Advance Praise for
PLAYING GOD

"I thoroughly enjoyed this book. Dr. Youn's unique insight will make you laugh, cry, shake your head, and recoil while wanting more."

—PAUL RUGGIERI, MD, author of *Confessions of a Surgeon*

"A riveting look at what it takes to become a premiere surgeon in today's wild west of medicine. Dr. Youn has written a moving and humorous memoir that is a must-read for medical students, doctors, and anyone interested in the fascinating world behind the clinic curtains and the operating room doors."

—DR. ANDREW ORDON, MD, FACS board-certified plastic surgeon and co-host of the Emmy Award-winning show, *The Doctors*

"Part *Botched*, part *Grey's Anatomy*, my good friend Dr. Tony Youn has written a fun and fascinating book that reveals what really happens behind the OR curtain. This is the rare medical memoir which doesn't take itself too seriously, but gives you the straight scoop on what it takes to become a top surgeon in today's crazy world of medicine. I loved it."

—DR. SANDRA LEE, aka "Dr. Pimple Popper," board-certified dermatologist and author of *Put Your Best Face Forward*

"In this well-written, heartfelt, and at times amusing book, Dr. Youn chronicles his journey towards a successful and fulfilling career as a plastic surgeon. The tribulations, joys, disappointments along the way, and the final triumph are all portrayed in a frank and humbling and sometimes humorous manner."

—FOAD NAHAI, MD, FACS, Professor of Surgery at Emory University School of Medicine, Editor-in-Chief of the *Aesthetic Surgery Journal*, Past President of the American Society for Aesthetic Plastic Surgery and the International Society of Aesthetic Plastic Surgery

"Dr. Youn has written a fascinating and informative book about the making of a surgeon. This gripping tale should be required reading for medical students and surgery residents."

—MATT MCCARTHY, MD, *New York Times* bestselling author of *Superbugs: The Race to Stop an Epidemic* and *The Real Doctor Will See You Shortly: A Physician's First Year*

"A must read! Dr. Youn details the arduous journey and rites of passage that all surgeons must endure. His humor and portrayal of life as a young doctor is the true reality of what it takes to become a caring and compassionate physician. Tony's transformation into a national physician leader and holistic plastic surgeon is proof that this journey was indeed worthwhile."

—ROD ROHRICH, MD, FACS, Founding Professor and Chair of the Department of Plastic Surgery, UT Southwestern Medical Center and Editor-in-Chief of the *Journal of Plastic and Reconstructive Surgery*

PLAYING GOD

PLAYING GOD

The Evolution of a Modern Surgeon

ANTHONY YOUN, M.D.
WITH ALAN EISENSTOCK

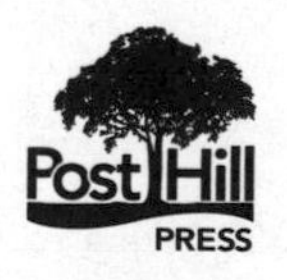

A POST HILL PRESS BOOK

Playing God:
The Evolution of a Modern Surgeon

ISBN: 978-1-64293-128-0
ISBN (eBook): 978-1-64293-129-7

Cover art by Cody Corcoran
Cover Photo by Justin McKee Photography
Author Photo by Seeger Studios
Interior design and composition, Greg Johnson, Textbook Perfect

All people, locations, events, and situations are portrayed to the best of the author's memory. While all of the events described are true, many names and identifying details have been changed to protect the privacy of the people involved.

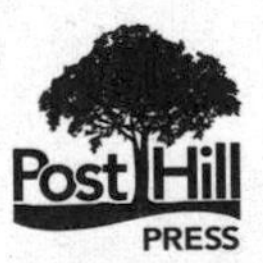

Post Hill Press
New York • Nashville
posthillpress.com
Published in the United States of America

This book is dedicated to my dad,
who always encouraged me to be
the best doctor I can be.

AUTHOR'S NOTE

This work is a memoir. I have changed names and some identifying details of many characters portrayed in this book—including all the doctors and patients—and a few individuals are composites. In some instances, the precise details, location, or timing of events have been changed to assist with the flow of the narrative and conceal the identities of those involved. Nevertheless, I believe this book provides an accurate portrait of my journey to become the doctor that I am today. I hope you enjoy it.

CONTENTS

PROLOGUE

See Twenty, Do a Hundred, Teach One

"My insides are falling out."

Ruth, forty-three, sits before me, her hospital gown covering her shockingly bulging belly. The contrast with her thin frame makes it look as if she's got a bowling ball tucked underneath.

"These past three years have been a nightmare," she says, quietly. "I was in a car accident. A drunk driver hit me. I was trapped in the car, against the steering wheel, for over an hour. They had to use the Jaws of Life to get me out. By then my spleen had burst. The doctors took it out, but then everything got infected. I had *seven* surgeries. My stomach is a complete mess. My insides are literally falling out."

She bites her lip and stares past me.

I don't just see Ruth's pain: I feel it. It's drawn all over her—from the double crease between her eyebrows to her slumped posture to the distinct aura of sadness pulsing off her.

Dr. Vivek Ramesh, tall, thin, a plastic surgery chief resident, stands next to me, his eyes glued on Ruth. In doctor training terms, Vivek is shadowing me. He shifts his weight, his eyes still fixed on Ruth. I can tell he's waiting for me to say something since I know he's never seen anything like this before.

"What do you mean, your insides are falling out?" I ask, gently.

"After they removed my spleen, I developed a terrible infection that kept me in the ICU for months," Ruth says. "By the time they got rid of the infection, my insides were so swollen they couldn't close up my abdomen. A plastic surgeon put a skin graft over my intestines. But they stick out. You can actually see them."

"Tell me...how does this affect your daily life?"

Her face reddens. "It's humiliating. People stop me and ask, 'When's the baby due?' And when I eat anything, even just a salad, my stomach sticks out even more. I can't go out in public. It's too embarrassing. I just stay home."

"Do you have pain?"

"Constantly. Sometimes I don't think I can take it anymore, but I refuse to take pain pills. I hate how they make me feel."

She lowers her head and studies the floor. Her voice drops to a whisper. "I look deformed. I've always prided myself on staying in shape, eating well. Then this happens. It wasn't even my fault."

She sniffles, swipes at a tear that slowly trickles down her cheek.

"And, um, my husband and me? Well, we can't...you know...I won't let him look at me unless I'm wearing a shirt or something. I don't really let him touch me. I'm afraid he'll feel my abdomen and get...disgusted."

Ruth raises her head. Her eyes have filled with tears.

"Please, Doctor Youn," she says. "Help me."

I can't imagine, I think. *How does this poor woman get through each day? How does she get through her life?*

I want so much to help her.

Please let me be able to help her.

This moment...this patient...this person...Ruth...is the reason I became a doctor.

I look into her eyes.

"Will you show the area to me, Ruth?" I say.

Ruth nods and lumbers over to the examination table. She pauses, exhales, and tries to hoist herself onto it, cradling her abdomen with one arm and grabbing the edge of the table with the other. She grunts, shakes her head, and looks at me, her eyes pleading. She can't lift herself. Vivek and I move swiftly to either side of her and help her onto the table. Then, settled, Ruth shudders, closes her eyes, and lifts her gown.

Her abdomen is littered with scars. In the middle lie her bowels covered with a nearly opaque layer of skin. I watch her intestines slowly move as spontaneous peristalsis occurs in waves, like large snakes slithering under a thin sheet.

Vivek's eyes pop open with shock.

I palpate Ruth's abdomen, trying to determine how much skin and muscle I may be able to mobilize to cover her exposed intestines. I sit before her for several seconds, staring at her abdomen, envisioning each step of the complicated surgery necessary to fix her. Suddenly, a comforting and familiar feeling sweeps through me. I feel a kind of calm. I know what to do. I then speak my favorite sentence in the English language:

"I can help you."

Ruth reaches over and grabs my hand. "Are you sure?"

I look into her eyes and smile, confidently, reassuringly.

"Yes," I say.

* * *

In the field of medicine, we have a saying: *see one, do one, teach one.*

I don't agree with this.

If physicians took this literally, we'd kill half our patients. I believe the saying should be: *see twenty, do a hundred, teach one.*

The surgery we'll be performing on Ruth—Vivek assisting—presents many similarities to a tummy tuck. Since Vivek has performed dozens of those, I decide to let him start.

"Scalpel, please," I say to the scrub technician, Christina. She places the scalpel in my hand. I turn it around, handle toward Vivek.

"OK, Vivek, make the incision."

He takes the knife, hesitates, and begins to cut along the line I drew on Ruth's abdomen. He incises through her skin with expert precision.

"Bovie cautery, please," I say to Christina.

She hands me the cautery device. I place it in Vivek's hand. "Dissect down toward the fascia."

He presses a button and the metal tip of the Bovie effortlessly glides through Ruth's underlying fat, bloodlessly splaying it open.

My eyes narrow.

Something doesn't look right.

"Stop," I say.

I move Vivek's hand away. The Bovie turns off.

"Do you see that?" I ask him.

"I...no...I...what do you mean?" Vivek's eyes, the only part of his face I can see above his mask, lock onto mine.

"Vivek," I say, "don't you see that loop of intestine?"

His pupils practically dilate. Sweat beads on his brow.

"My God, I was two seconds away from cutting right into it."

A single loop of small intestine, the width of a pinky finger, lies scarred and adhered to the overlying skin. In a "normal" person, this intestine would lie in a completely different position. But Ruth isn't normal. Her previous surgeries and infections have caused her insides to no longer conform to any anatomy textbook. Cutting open her intestine in a nonintestinal operation would be a total disaster. Ruth would have come in for a tummy tuck and left with a colostomy bag. Or, worst-case scenario, in a body bag.

I gently place my gloved hand on Vivek's. "It's all right."

I take over for Vivek, who stands to the side, immobile as a statue, except for his hands, which begin to tremble.

I complete the rest of the surgery. It takes three hours. I keep Ruth's intestines intact and put them inside her, where they belong. And I flatten her stomach.

After I insert the last stitch, Vivek and I take off our gowns and gloves.

"You OK, Vivek?" I say.

"I think so." He slowly shakes his head. "I'm still reeling from almost botching the whole operation."

"You didn't botch it. It was a learning experience. I promise you, remembering this case will make you a better surgeon."

"I guess you learn more from your mistakes than from your successes."

"Absolutely. Especially in surgery." I touch Vivek's arm. "You're going to be OK."

I want to encourage him. No. I *need* to encourage him. Suddenly, I see myself as Vivek, a young, inexperienced, unsure resident. I remember how much I needed encouragement, especially after I'd made a mistake, when I felt I was flailing.

As if he's reading my mind, Vivek says, "Doctor Youn, did you ever doubt yourself? Did you wonder if you'd ever become as good as the doctors who trained you?"

I grin at Vivek. "When I was a resident, I was the king of self-doubt. Even *after* residency. Man, do I have stories."

* * *

Doctors don't become good surgeons overnight. The ability to remove a tumor, fix a heart, or reconstruct a breast doesn't happen over a span of hours, or days, or weeks, or even months. Neither does the ability to gain the trust of frightened patients and give them hope. But with enough persistence and compassion even doctors-in-training who initially lack confidence and skill can become excellent surgeons.

When I graduated from medical school, I didn't have a clue what it meant to be a real doctor. I knew what I'd learned from textbooks. But textbook knowledge means little in an actual hospital. It took me the entire six years after medical school, working and training as a resident, taking care of the sick, the injured, and even the hopeless, to become a qualified doctor and a competent surgeon.

My journey didn't end there. My education continued into the early stages of practice. In fact, it was during those years, after I became a legitimate board-certified plastic and reconstructive surgeon, that I questioned myself the most. They say a little knowledge is a dangerous thing. In medicine, it can be a deadly thing.

I often worried that I wasn't good enough. I was terrified that I would be the anti-Hippocrates: that I would first do harm. I sent many desperate pleas to God to intervene in my patients' well-being. Thankfully, those moments were tempered and balanced by times that I made my patients' lives healthier. Not just healthier, but happier. Better.

My personal journey of self-doubt, questioning, and learning reflects a path that most surgeons—most doctors—experience, each in their own way. While the following is my personal story, aspects of it apply to all surgeons, even all doctors. Hopefully, for every physician, these successes and failures will culminate in one common result.

Becoming a good doctor.

* * *

Several months later.

I'm vacationing with my wife and kids on the west coast of Michigan, at Grand Haven, my old stomping grounds.

It's a sunny day with a low breeze. The muggy ninety-degree Michigan heat simmers while a beach band plays in the distance. The sounds of seagulls squawking as they search for food and kids laughing and shouting as they frolic in the water bring me back to my days as a resident physician. Dozens of evenings I moonlighted as a musician in this town, playing guitar and singing "Margaritaville" in tiki bars. Then, exhausted yet exhilarated, I'd head back to Grand Rapids, put on my doctor costume and my serious surgeon face, and pray that I knew what I was doing at the hospital the next morning—or at least that I could fake it until I figured it out.

This day, as I sit on the beach, the faces of patients and their families fill my memory. I see faces that plead for help, long for comfort, cry with grief, and smile with gratitude. These are the faces of the patients who allowed me to be their doctor, their surgeon. These are the faces to whom I owe my career.

The images shimmy, blur, and blend away. I turn and focus on a mom in a one-piece bathing suit playing with her children near the water. There's something familiar about her. I watch her run through the waves, chasing three little boys, none older than five or six years. Laughing and splashing, they fall into the shallow tide together.

Then I realize why she looks familiar.

The woman is Ruth.

I watch her enjoying this beautiful day with her kids. I spot her husband sitting on a blanket several yards away, grinning at his lovely wife and beautiful children.

Ruth glances my way. She does a double take, and then she stares at me. A moment later, she waves.

I wave back.

She points to her kids, her husband, and her stomach.

And then she smiles.

All the doubts, insecurities, and nearly ruptured intestines fade away.

In that moment, I know it is all worthwhile.

I smile back.

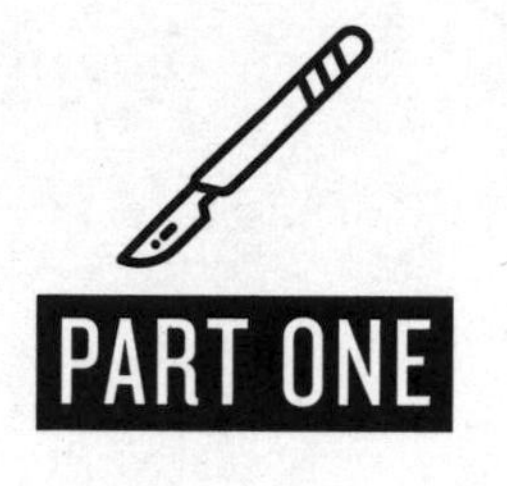

PART ONE

INTERNSHIP

1

Putting Out Fires

I am a doctor.

Every time I say that to myself, an aftershock of happiness ripples through me, 10.0 on the Richter scale.

Even though at times it seemed like this moment would never come to pass, I have finally, blessedly, put medical school in my rearview mirror.

I have triumphed. I have slayed the dragon of sleepless nights, endless exams, cadaver dissections, "practice" physical exams, bossy physicians and nurses, and several oceans of paperwork.

I am a doctor.

Starting tomorrow, July 1, I will be a first-year resident, commonly known as an intern.

I have been blessed with the perfect girlfriend, Amy, who's finishing medical school here in Grand Rapids. She has one year left to go before beginning a pediatrics residency. We're going strong. That is, in the ten- to fifteen-minute increments we get to spend with each other, when we're actually awake. She's so busy and exhausted that when we catch a rare evening together, we order in food and rent a movie. Twelve minutes into the movie, like clockwork, she's out cold and I get to watch her sleep. Which is great. She's so beautiful when she sleeps, mouth slightly open, purring like a kitten. So cute. There she is, passed out, cuddled into me, her brown hair brushing my cheek. I get to spend the next two hours trying to get the feeling back in my arm and shoulder.

And now that I'm a doctor, I have done what every doctor dreams of doing once they're finally done climbing out of Dante's Circles of Hell, commonly known as medical school. I bought a hot new car. Well, OK, a hot *used* car. But to me it's new. And totally hot. A snazzy Toyota RAV4 to replace my ancient, rusted-out, held-together-by-chewing-gum-and-baling-wire Ford Tempo. That infuriating twenty-four-seven pinging noise that drowned out the radio and ground away on the last good nerve I had? Turned out to be a death rattle. The Ford Tempo bit the dust, bought the farm, and moved on to that great auto showroom in the sky. I slide behind the wheel of my RAV4 confident that I can finally attain a speed of over thirty-five on the freeway without my molars coming loose.

Most important, though, I've earned the respect of my old-country Korean parents. Especially my dad, a doctor himself. A man of few words, he was moved to deliver the following stirring words of encouragement while slurping my mother's squid soup and chewing a spoonful of tentacles: "Tony, OK, you be plastic surgeon, OK. Not as good as transplant surgeon, or neurosurgeon, or trauma surgeon. Why you not be transplant surgeon? Good money. Best money. But at least plastic surgeon much better than pediatrician or, God forbid, family doctor. Make lots more money. But be careful. Be like Daddy. Thirty years ob-gyn, Daddy never get sued. Never. Not once. Don't get sued! Good soup."

Smile. Slurp. Swallow.

Of course, to be fair, on the downside, I owe $125,000 in loans.

Let me repeat that—$125,000.

And I'm about to go further into debt. I will pay all that off once I complete the next leg of my journey, which starts tomorrow. A five-year residency: three years of general surgery, followed by two years of plastic surgery. On top of twenty years of school already? That means by the time I'm done, I will have spent 80 percent of my life in school. No worries. Par for the course. That's how we doctors roll.

Speaking of worries. While I've been accepted into Michigan State's program in Grand Rapids, I admit, OK, I'm having massive opening day jitters. Because, when my brain asks me, *What could go wrong?* I have to answer: *Everything*. Look, when you're a professional baseball player and you strike out with the bases loaded in the bottom of the ninth, your team loses. When you strike out as a doctor, people go brain-dead, their organs fail, and yes, sometimes they die.

I have to swat those away. And I will because—

I am a doctor.

Right?

* * *

Like gunslingers emerging from a mist, we stride together in slow motion, the five of us, flanked side by side, ready to do battle with everything from necrotic gallbladders to perforated intestines to punctured lungs. Nurses and administrative staff retreat, allowing us to pass. We take up the entire hallway. We bash through the saloon doors at the end of the corridor. We wear white. Our starched, unblemished, *long* white coats glide across the linoleum. Our heads are held high, our eyes are unblinking, intelligent, focused, fearless, the color of cement. We are first-year residents. We are the law.

We are...*lost*.

Totally, completely, stupidly lost.

At least that's how I feel, though I would never say it to *anyone*.

The gunslinger image lasts maybe five seconds before real time—real life—sets in.

We are in fact five interns breaking for lunch after a two-hour orientation session where we learned the basics of CPR, practicing first aid on EMT dummies, and then, for some of us, on real live dummies: each other. I came this close to giving mouth-to-mouth to a nerdy bespectacled musky-smelling guy named Conrad, until someone stepped in and saved my bacon. We have officially been practicing doctors for all of three hours.

Even after orientation activities, we remain an improv troupe—ready to wing it in medical emergencies, clueless in the heat of the moment, as everyone yells out suggestions of what to inject, cut off, or cut into. We are sometimes all that stands between a patient slipping from the hospital ward down into the basement morgue. Which is just as horrifying as it sounds. But you probably couldn't tell from just looking at us. We give the illusion of being actual, real, seasoned, competent doctors. Operative word being "illusion." There are no "Doctor-in-Training" signs on our backs, like those signs you see in cars where terrified teenagers are trying to learn to drive. You know, the ones you steer as far away from as possible.

We enter the cafeteria, the smell of boiled cabbage laced with disinfectant causing a momentary gag reflex. We slither single file into the food line and watch happy people in hairnets ladle thick steaming brown murky blobby globs into bowls and, snickering, hand them to us. We sidestep to the end, gather forks, spoons, napkins, and commandeer a sticky table in the far corner. We smell, taste, and chew, tentatively. Finally, Jessica, short, thin, and Asian, speaks for all of us. "Yum."

Shelley sits across from me, husky voice and Vampira looks. She's a gunner I know from medical school, so-called because of her frenetic pace and kill-at-all-costs/leave-no-survivors world view, driving full speed ahead toward becoming a trauma surgeon. She pushes her bowl away like it's radioactive (which it might well be) and says, "I was reading the General Surgery Residency manual last night..."

"Wait," Jessica stares at her. "You were reading what?"

"She reads manuals like that for fun," I say. "Insurance policies, warranties. Turns her on. To her they're like porn." I slurp the stew. Or the liquid mulch. Or whatever the hell it is. It's not terrible. Hell, I lived on five-dollar pizzas and Burger King for four years in medical school.

"Enjoy your light reading," Jessica sniffs. "I'm more hands-on. Like to roll up my sleeves, get dirty."

"I hear you," Conrad says, his eyes half closed. "I love the smell of human flesh getting cauterized."

"I know. There's nothing like the smell of napalm in the morning, right?" Jessica says.

"Exactly," Conrad says, eyes still glazed.

"You're serious," Jessica says. After a pause, she turns to me. "He's serious."

Conrad shrugs. "I like the smell of burning flesh. Something about it. Relaxes me."

"We have a winner," Jessica says.

"Where's Garth?" Gunner Shelley asks, scanning the cafeteria. "He was right behind us in line, and then he disappeared."

"He does that," Conrad says.

On cue, Garth Ellington's laugh, a deep, booming roar, cuts through the ambient murmuring in the cafeteria. Then Garth appears at the edge of our table with the general surgery chief resident, Dr. Weinberger, a tall, balding *macher* at the hospital. He throws his head back in what seems to me an over-the-top, theatrical laugh, then leans a hand on Dr. Weinberger's shoulder.

"I never heard that one," Garth says, and repeats the punch line: "*Either way you're screwed!*" The two of them laugh again.

"Don't forget," Dr. Weinberger says, with a grin like Heath Ledger's Joker. "We tee off tomorrow morning, seven thirty sharp."

"Put my clubs in the car this morning," Garth says.

Then, looking at me, Dr. Weinberger says, "Because if you're on call, Garth, I'm sure I can convince somebody to switch with you...."

"No, no, I'm fine. I wouldn't want to inconvenience anyone."

"OK, then. And, oh, Saturday, it's three for cocktails."

"I'm looking forward to that. I haven't done much sailing."

"You'll take to it, I can tell...*like a fish to water....*"

Garth and Dr. Weinberger howl like a couple of wasted frat boys.

"What the *hell*?" Jessica says to me, low.

More laughing. Slapping of backs. Dr. Weinberger makes a pistol with his thumb and index finger, and "shoots" Garth. He gives a dismissive sneer toward the rest of us, *scut monkeys all*, his dark expression says, and bounds off toward the swinging doors leading out of the cafeteria.

"Sorry, guys," Garth says, vaulting onto a chair at the head of the table. He lowers his head and actually blushes. "He cornered me."

"Golf? Cocktails? Sailing? Maybe it's me." I pretend to sniff my underarms. "No. I'm good. So, Garth, what *was* that?"

Garth shrugs as he extracts a Power Bar from his shirt pocket, unwrapping and nibbling with small dainty bites. "I don't know. Weiney has been very nice to me."

"*Weiney?*" all of us spout, in chorus.

Garth lowers his head, reddens, and chuckles.

I'd known about and competed against Garth Ellington since I listed Grand Rapids as my first choice for residency a few months earlier. Dr. Karr, a dean at the medical school, warned me that while I was a good candidate, he considered me a long shot to get in. Grand Rapids had exactly two open spots in plastic surgery and they'd already committed one to Garth. Not that Garth was ever an actual, active rival. He just happened to be kind of in my way. And I kind of got it. He overshadowed me. To be honest, he overshadowed everybody, the way James Bond overshadows all other mortals. Garth was older, established, and not a punk like the rest of us. He was thirty-three, married, father of two adorable, precocious kids, a black belt in kung fu, a gourmet cook, an amateur sculptor, a scratch golfer, a young Patrick Dempsey lookalike, a gifted doctor with maestro's hands, and worst of all, he appeared to be genuinely modest, polite, generous, and kind. He entered elevators last, asked everyone their floor, and operated all the buttons like a doorman. He helped elderly people cross the street. He handed out five-dollar bills to the homeless. He shoveled his neighbors' sidewalks and driveways in winter and mowed their lawns in summer. If he washed his car, he washed yours too. And in his spare time, I'm pretty sure he saved orphans and puppies.

You could easily hate him.

I don't.

I like him, I enjoy his company, and, even though I shouldn't, I envy his luck.

Hell, I want to *be* him when I grow up.

"You know, Garth," Gunner Shelley says, pursing her lips, crossing her legs and swinging them slowly, back and forth, back and forth, twirling a few strands of hair between two fingers flashing bloodred nail polish, "I was studying the General Surgery Residency manual last night in *bed*..."

"Me too!" Garth says, perking up, carefully sweeping a few straggling crumbs of Power Bar into his palm. "Wealth of information in there. And surprisingly well written."

"Shoot me," Jessica says, eyes rolling.

Garth's cell phone rings, his ringtone the jarring overloud tinkling chorus to "I Just Can't Wait to Be King" from *The Lion King*. Another Garth shrug. "My kids picked it," he whispers apologetically, then changes his tone into a melodious singsong baritone and croons into the phone, "Doctor Ellington."

"Gag," Jessica mutters.

"Uh-huh," Garth says. "Oh, absolutely, I'd be honored. Yes, oh, yes. Very excited, Weiney, *very* excited. I'll go right over and scrub up and join you in a few in the OR. No. Thank *you*."

He folds his phone closed. He feels the heat of our stares on his neck. "That was, um, Weiney, ah, Doctor Weinberger. No big deal. I'm going to assist him on a gall bladder removal...."

"*Today?*" Shelley's face pulses an alarming shade of purple, in most humans a sign of distress. In her case, the sign of a flat-out pissed-off subtitle reading: *Why does Garth get preferential treatment and I'm stuck with these freaks?* "We just finished orien-ta-*tion*. Everyone tells me that for the next two weeks we'll be lucky to hold a *clamp*."

"I don't get it either." Garth's arms splay across the table helplessly. "Catch up with you guys later? Maybe grab a beer? Oh, I can't tonight. I'm making moussaka. Rain check?"

He tosses this invitation over his shoulder as he sprints out of the cafeteria, flicking his Power Bar crumbs into the waste receptacle by the exit, waving at us, and then lowering his shoulder into the saloon doors.

"Doesn't matter," Shelley sniffs, gathering her stuff. "In a few years, I'll be doing trauma surgery while he's doing boob jobs. No offense, Tony."

"None taken," I say, too numb to feel offended. Or to feel anything.

"I give him credit," Shelley says, standing abruptly, nearly tipping over the table. "You see an opening, you go for it. Plus, I like the guy. Who doesn't? And he's kinda hot."

"Ever notice the way blood pools up from a knife wound?" Conrad says, his eyes still half closed. "The patterns that form? Very modernistic. Beautiful. Evocative."

A moment later, the others gone, Jessica and I sit at the table, saying nothing, feeling, in my case, stunned, overwhelmed, overmatched, underprepared, out of place, and brutally alone.

"You and me, Tone," she says, finally. "Looks like we better stick together."

"Because we're Asian?" I drone.

She stares at me. "No, fool, because we're *normal.*"

* * *

I walk the halls of the hospital alone, my mood swinging like a pendulum on steroids from excitement to confusion back to excitement, then to anxiety, back to excitement, then on to anxiety, anxiety, and more anxiety. Life is now a panic attack waiting to happen.

Images from my third year of medical school, my first clinical rotation, internal medicine, flood over me, a grainy black-and-white movie trapped in my brain. As on that first day two years ago, I'm once again rendered momentarily mute. The sounds now here—the beeping, whirring, moaning, phones ringing, jarring voice-overs from overhead speakers, footsteps swishing—swamp me. Smells descend like falling snow and stick, a metallic mint mixed with something vaguely chemical, and a little sour death under it all. I shiver. The air feels chillier than I remember. Unseasonably cold.

"Your job," a resident said at orientation that morning, "is putting out fires." He paused and added, "Not to start them."

Big, uncomfortable laugh.

I turn a corner, slow my pace, halt.

I lean into a wall, close my eyes, and breathe.

It takes only a moment before a new wave blows over me.

An awareness.

An adrenaline rush.

I'm here, I say to myself, *because I belong.*

I open my eyes and push off the wall.

I'm ready.

I'm a doctor.

* * *

The day expands.

We go from twenty-four hours with sustained patches of daylight and variations of weather and temperature ending with at least some time blocked out for sleep, to thirty-six hours straight of climate-controlled night in a zombie state.

Every day I arrive at six a.m. and round on the patients on the floor. I caffeinate, recaffeinate, and wipe sleep from my eyes as I check charts, go over what the medical student has written previously, correct or sign off on that. Then at seven thirty I gather with the other interns for breakfast while the residents do their rounds. After breakfast, we get our assignments for the day. Dr. Weinberger, usually the chief resident in charge, hands us all surgeries. For now, only temporarily he assures us, we will assist, observe, and fill out the necessary paperwork. I swear I catch him winking at Garth. Rumor has it, he's already completed a gallbladder removal and an appendectomy. On his own! I know this: when we invite him to join us for dinner at our local Subway, he begs off because of a previous engagement. He's the only one of us who's been invited to a get-to-know-the-residents dinner at the 1913 Room. *The* legendary Grand Rapids steakhouse. I wonder how, in less than twenty-four hours, I went from being a promising resident to a giant loser, with a capital L right in the middle of my forehead.

After he drops this news on us at breakfast, he shrugs apologetically, and then slips away.

"Heard he's the copilot on a colon removal," Gunner Shelley says, more in awe than in envy.

"And we'll be lucky if we are allowed to dig our fingers into a moist body cavity and get blood on our gloves," Conrad says, practically spitting the words out. Then feeling caught in the glare of our stares, he says, "What?"

* * *

Day two.

My first procedure.

I am to assist on a breast biopsy. The surgeon, Dr. Bledsoe, is a tall, severe-looking man with a lantern jaw. I will write up the mountain of paperwork and help in any way I can. Which at this point will be trying not to drop any Junior Mints into the patient once she's opened. We scrub up together, Dr. Bledsoe and I, two doctors, colleagues, allegedly, although he never speaks to me or even attempts eye contact. We begin the procedure. Dr. Bledsoe stands, motionless, for what feels like an hour. He looks like one of those mimes in the mall. My hands begin to tremble. My palms start to sweat. Finally, Dr. Bledsoe swivels his lantern face toward me, his eyes smoking in some kind of Vulcan death ray.

"Well?" he snaps.

"Yes?"

"Get started."

I blink rapidly. "Oh, OK, get...*started*?"

As if it has its own little built-in brain, my hand shoots out and grabs the closest instrument in the vicinity. A clamp. I watch my hand bring it to me and hold it against my chest.

"What the hell are you going to do with *that*?" Dr. Bledsoe says in a puffed-out, breathy voice. He's Darth Vader in scrubs.

"I have no idea what the hell I'm doing. Seriously, no idea at all. Please don't make me do this. I beg you. Just let me watch a little until I get the hang of it."

That's what I feel like saying. This is what I say instead:

"I...well...I'm not...me?"

Dr. Bledsoe hisses, "Put that down and pick up a knife."

I think I hear him add in a low voice "you idiot." But I may be hallucinating.

"A...knife?" I say it as if I'm unfamiliar with the term. I put the clamp aside. I grab the nearest knife, a gleaming scalpel. "Watch out, I've got a knife!" I force a smile under my mask.

Nobody laughs. Nobody says anything.

"Give it to me!" He yanks the scalpel out of my hand. Then, voice suddenly all nasally and dripping with sarcasm, "*Thank* you, Doctor Youn." Well, at least he knows my name.

He cuts. I watch. We don't speak. I scarcely breathe. Later, my hands still shaking, I dive in and do his paperwork, which for the moment becomes my specialization.

I find me asking myself, am I really a doctor?

* * *

Over the next couple of weeks, our gang of five bonds, mostly over breakfast, all of us struggling to find our way. All of us except Garth, of course, who has apparently entered his first-year residency as the bright, shining star of the universe. The rest of us spend our days mistaking clamps for scalpels, rounding on patients and filling out paperwork, praying to be invited to participate in even one second of a surgery, any kind of surgery. Garth, on the other hand, assists Dr. Weinberger and Dr. Bledsoe in appendectomies and gallbladder removals, repairs hernias, cuts off colons, and on the weekends plays golf, sails, and parties with the surgeons.

One morning, Conrad, eyes half shut, nostrils flaring, blurts, "I'm so sick of this. I want to cut some flesh. I want to dip my hands into some blood!"

In an inadvertent call and response, I blurt right back, "I actually agree with you. Cut flesh. Dip hands in blood."

"Patience, children," Jessica says. "Every journey begins with a single step." She looks at our stunned faces. "Too Zen?"

Another thirty-six-hour shift follows. Still no action.

* * *

Three a.m.

Dozing in the call room, I answer a page. ER calling. A man has arrived with searing pain in his lower right quadrant.

Appendicitis, I think. *Without a doubt.*

Two reasons.

One: searing pain in the lower right quadrant almost always indicates appendicitis.

Two: appendicitis almost always occurs at three a.m.

Book it.

I begin the paperwork. I order a CT scan. I fill out more paperwork. The CT scan comes back.

Appendicitis.

My total time expenditure so far: two hours, fifteen minutes.

I call Dr. Bledsoe.

"Hey, it's Tony. There's an appendicitis in the ER."

"OK." A loud, gaping yawn. "Do the consents and call me when they go to surgery."

"Got it."

Consents signed. More paperwork. Another hour. I call Bledsoe.

"Hey, it's Tony again. That appendicitis is going into surgery."

"On my way."

Through the phone I hear the clatter of a fork scraping a plate, a slurp of coffee. My mind wanders. I can almost smell a breakfast of freshly squeezed orange juice, pancakes with melted butter and warm maple syrup, a cup of fresh hot coffee. My mouth waters. I look at the half-eaten Snickers in my hand. I toss it in the trash. I'm slapped back to reality.

Bledsoe arrives. He performs the appendectomy. I stand by like a department store dummy dressed as a doctor. One highlight. At the midway point I hand him a knife. He receives it with a low, appreciative "ha" from under his mask. And for the first time he makes eye contact. I detect a slight collegial nod. I think maybe, just maybe, he'll let me tie off the appendix. No such luck. Dr. Bledsoe completes the whole operation himself. By my watch, the procedure takes thirty-one minutes. Finished, he pulls off his mask. "OK, write it up."

He leaves. I complete the paperwork.

Total time I invested with this patient: five hours.

Total time Dr. Bledsoe invested with this patient: thirty-one minutes.

Total number of hours Bledsoe got to sleep: seven hours.

Total number of hours I got to sleep: zero.

Normally, I would almost certainly be bitter, anxious, or angry. But I'm not. I'm just antsy, sick of sitting on the bench. Put me in, Coach! I'm ready to play.

I determine after the appendectomy to approach each surgery as an opportunity, embrace whatever task I'm given, and be grateful, no matter how small or insignificant my role. I know Jessica is right. I simply have to be patient. My time will come.

About a week later, my patience pays off.

* * *

A Monday after breakfast.

Dr. Weinberger distributes the day's surgeries. I listen casually, trying to tamp down any expectations, especially when he looks over his list and says to the Great and Glorious Garth, "Hey, you know what, Garth? Why don't you do the gallbladder? You can assist me. I'll tell you what. Even better. I'll hold the camera. You play the lead."

At our table, the five of us huddled. Gunner Shelley shifts in her chair and swears under her breath. Conrad lowers his head and digs a finger into his ear. Jess and I share a look somewhere between give up and awestruck, with a tiny bit of let's-slip-some-arsenic-in-Garth's protein bar mixed in.

Great, I think, *sweet. Another freaking gallbladder, his third, or fourth. I've lost count, and this one he's basically doing on his own. The surgeon will be the backup. I haven't even done one surgery yet. Not one...*

"Let's see, who's left?" Weinberger says. "Tony. OK, hmm. What do I have for you? You know what? Time for you to jump in."

I blink. I can't believe it. Today's the day. A menu of surgeries passes before my eyes. Appendectomy. Colectomy. A gallbladder of my very own. Or—dare I even hope?—I'll be assisting on an eight-hour whipple, the most intense, difficult, and prestigious surgery that can be done. *You're tripping, Tony. Take it easy, Tony. Don't be greedy.*

"Big Tony, you're going to do the pilonidal cyst."

"The what now? Did you say the pilonidal cyst?"

"That's what I said. A jeep seat. An ass boil. Enjoy."

Do I hear...snickering?

Is that what I hear?

Freaking *snickering*?

I look up and catch Conrad, Jessica, and Shelley looking at each other, trying not to burst out in evil laughter.

"If you need any help," Shelley says, "ask Conrad. He's the closest thing we have to an ass here."

I stand, tower over the group, draw myself up, and smile. "They always say it's best to start at the bottom."

They laugh, all of them.

This time as I head out, each one slaps my palm.

* * *

I see nothing but ass, ass, and more ass.

The immense, obese, hairy ass of Carmine Mondelo, a 350-pound forklift operator. It's like getting mooned by Chewbacca. And inside Carmine's immense, jiggling, hairy rear end sits a cyst the size of a golf ball.

I freeze in the doorway.

I don't know if it's from lack of sleep or downing gobs of candy bars and straight shots of Coke and coffee, but the room seems distorted. I feel as if I'm looking in a fun-house mirror. The walls tilt, shimmer, shimmy, and close in. The ceiling rips off and sails away, and the walls collapse. The cyst inside Carmine's butt grows, becoming the size of a grapefruit, then a basketball, then a large rock, then a larger rock, and, finally, a giant, jagged, steaming ass-boulder. I flash on the cyst rolling toward me, crushing me, trapping me, flattening me. I imagine my death certificate. Cause of death: ass cyst.

A hand—The nurse's? The resident's? Dr. Rabuchin's?—slathers brown antiseptic all over Carmine's fleshy thighs and flabby butt and swabs the cyst itself. A deep bass, like the voice of God, descends from above, shaking the earth:

"All right, Tony, start cutting."

I snap back to reality.

It's not God. Not even close. It's Dr. Rabuchin, a white-haired old-timer in his early seventies, on the fast track toward retirement, smiling kindly behind wire rims with lenses thick as a hockey rink. I drift into the room and find a table full of scalpels.

"Take it slow," Dr. Rabuchin says.

"Hurry it *up,*" Carmine wails.

I choose a scalpel. I consider the cyst. The knife seems woefully inadequate. I choose a much bigger blade. I assume my position over his derriere, preparing to dig out the disgusting cyst. One thing I know for sure, I can't miss. I press the big-boy scalpel into the cyst. It's hard as granite.

"A little more oomph," Dr. Rabuchin says.

I manage to refrain from telling him how incredibly helpful his comment is. I shake my head, exhale, lean between the cheeks, and cut again, applying more elbow grease. The cyst bursts. A volcanic eruption of yellowish-brown pus blasts out of Carmine's butt and spews ass-lava all over my face.

"AGHGHGGHGH!" Carmine wails.

"AGHGHGGHGH!" I blurt out.

I wipe away the ooze from the lenses of my surgical goggles with a gloved hand. It smells like death. I take a second to gather myself and realize what is actually going on. I'm a surgeon with a blade in my hand and I'm expected to cut.

It's my time. I've unsheathed my Samurai sword.

I move in. Looking through yellow-caked plastic lenses, I dice, chop, and slice away at that pilonidal cyst with the swashbuckling swagger of a Japanese cyst ninja.

"Nice work," Dr. Rabuchin says. "Clean. Well, except for your face."

I blink and nod.

Then, through my curtain of wet yellowish-brown goo, my face blossoms into a giant grin. I have begun. No...I have arrived.

Hello, Dr.Youn.

* * *

I become Dr. Rabuchin's main man.

I graduate from cutting out pilonidal cysts to stripping veins, a sometimes tricky and always bloody procedure that gives me my first small taste of plastic surgery. Women after pregnancy or entering menopause, or people who gain a significant amount of weight, are prime candidates to get puffy purple veins, known as varicose veins. These veins cannot only look unsightly, but also cause pain and even ulcerate. One way to treat a varicose vein is surgically. You begin by marking the spot you want to treat on the patient with a Sharpie. Then, according to your mark, you make an incision over the vein, slice open the area, clamp it, yank out the vein and quickly stitch the area closed. You have to move fast because you've pulled out a freaking *vein* and blood will *gush*.

We're talking major bleeding. White water rapids of blood. A real-life Quentin Tarantino film.

Dr. Rabuchin supervises my first vein stripping. He likes to watch. A little too much. He measures and marks the spot on the patient's leg—a nice woman in her fifties—and then stands back on the sidelines and provides encouraging running commentary as I cut. Commentary that is painfully willie inducing.

"You got it, Tony. See that vein. Grab that clamp. Now *take* that vein. Yank it out! Yank hard! It's coming! Oh, baby, yeah, it's coming! Beautiful! It's a geyser! Now stitch it fast. Fast, Tony! Magnificent!" His eyes roll up and back. He screams, "It's like rapture!"

After my second vein stripping, with Dr. Rabuchin observing, consulting, and doing his creepy cheering, he allows me to do my third vein stripping while he huddles silently at the door. Convinced I've got the hang of it, he assigns me a vein stripping several mornings a week and hardly shows up for the procedures. I'm basically on my own.

I love it.

Love. It.

I'm not only working with my hands, but I can see the results of my work. My vein stripping makes these people's legs look better—tighter, no lumps, and no trace of that nasty prune color. Even better, the patients are more comfortable and seem genuinely happy with the work I've done. For the first time, I get a hint of how I might feel after I will—in the far distant future—perform appearance-altering plastic surgery. The feeling that by improving a person's appearance, I have actually improved that person's life.

In the meantime, I work my on-again, off-again thirty-six-hour shifts. I take the exhaustion and discomfort in stride. The workload comes with the territory. It's part of the job. Looking back, I'm amazed by what humans can get used to.

* * *

Two thirty a.m.

The on-call nurse wakes me to check a patient's breathing. I bound off my wafer-thin mattress, the springs taking a bite out of my back, and whistle as I walk down the corridor toward the patient's room. "It's two thirty in the morning," the nurse grumbles. "Why are you in such a good mood? Hell, you're always in a good mood. Frankly, it's annoying."

"Sorry," I say. "It's this job."

The nurse looks at me, confused and possibly concerned that I may soon become a danger to myself and others.

"Look, I've had two other jobs in my life," I say. "I was a waiter at a Pizza Hut, and I ground up paprika in a spice factory. Believe it or not, being a doctor is way better. Although I got all my pizzas at half price and all-you-can-eat paprika."

"I'm gonna tell you a secret, Doctor Youn," the nurse says. "We always hope you're the doc on call."

"Really? You just made my night!" I say giddily. My love, respect, and reliance on nurses begins that night, early in my first year of residency.

It continues to this day.

2

The One That Stays with Me

It's said that every doctor has a handful of patients whom he or she remembers forever. Even though we might see thousands of patients over our careers, most of their names and faces blend into a pastiche of colors, genders, conditions, and outcomes. But there are always those few that stick in our heads—or, more accurately, haunt us for the rest of our lives.

This is one of mine.

One morning, I get a page from Weiney, Dr. Weinberger, Chief Resident. He wants me to head down to the ER to evaluate a new consultation for the general surgery service. Nothing out of the ordinary here, totally generic, exactly like hundreds of other pages I get as a surgeon-in-training.

The ER doc greets me the moment I walk through the sliding door, his face a deathly shade of white. His urgency and his pallor are both totally out of the ordinary. He rushes toward me, encroaching into my personal space. He's so close I can identify his cologne. Hugo Boss.

"Tony. Very glad you're here," he says. Then he lowers his voice to a whisper. "I have to warn you, I've never seen anything like this. It's...I mean...I don't even..."

My heart starts to race. "What is it?"

"I don't want you to freak out in front of the patient." He takes me aside to a corner, standing so close my eyes begin tearing from his cologne.

"What's going on?"

"Well, it's...this woman...her breast...it's..." He leans in even closer, so close his lips are practically touching my ear. "Eaten away."

I pull back, confused. "Eaten away? What do you mean? Was she attacked by a wild animal or something?"

He hands me her chart. "You just have to see it. It's so sad." He lets out a deep sigh. "Just don't freak out when you see it."

It might just be me, but when I'm told not to freak out, my brain immediately begins to freak out. I can't stop imagining the horror I'm about to see. A breast torn apart by dog teeth? Chest flesh gnawed away? Nipple chewed off?

I study her chart.

Sandra. Sixty years old. Married. Kids. Grandkids. Farming family from Gowen, Michigan, a tiny village near my old hometown in Greenville. Farm country in the middle of the boondocks. I scan her history. No other known medical problems. Family physician is deceased.

I take a deep breath, knock on her door, walk in, and introduce myself.

A mildly overweight woman sits on the exam table. Her husband sits in the chair beside her, holding her hand. A loose hospital gown covers everything but her ankles and hospital-issued gray socks. She looks older than her sixty years, with dark circles under her eyes and stringy gray hair down to her shoulders. Although she appears like any other patient seeing a doctor for a routine visit, something exudes from her, a sense that I've never seen before and that I will never forget.

She exudes—fear.

Primal fear.

She looks scared to death.

I want to jump right in. I want to fix whatever is causing her crippling fear. That's my instinct. But I allow my training to take over. Four years of medical school taught me first and foremost to put the patient at ease by developing a rapport. Start by getting to know her—*then* begin to solve the problem.

So, I start to talk. I tell Sandra how I grew up in Greenville. I ask her what high school her kids went to, where she goes to church. Her shoulders drop from being up around her ears and return to their normal position. Everything unclenches. Her expression softens. She even smiles.

Then I ask her what's going on with her breast.

She looks down at the ground as she talks, deep embarrassment cloaking her.

Her words come out haltingly, slowly, deliberately. "For the past two years I've had a problem with my right breast," she says. "It started as a small lump, just under the skin, but it's gotten bigger and bigger. About a year ago it started oozing, so over the last couple months I've been putting a diaper over the area. I change it twice a day. I think there might be something wrong though. It smells really bad."

I turn to her husband. "Have you seen it?"

"No," her husband says, his voice low, gruff. "She won't let me look at it."

I turn back to Sandra. "Would you mind if I take a peek?"

She keeps her eyes focused on the ground, lets out a soft sigh, and nods. She hesitates, then pulls up her hospital gown and unclasps her bra. When she removes the bra, I see a diaper stuck to her right breast. She looks over at her husband. "Turn around," she says. "Don't look."

He grunts and shifts his body away from her. Sandra sighs again and then slowly removes the diaper.

It takes everything in my power not to gasp out loud.

The right breast has been completely obliterated. Nipple. Areola. Breast mound. All gone.

Lumpy flesh that looks like pus-yellow oatmeal clings to her completely flat chest.

The smell wallops me. I've never smelled anything like it before or since. It seems to seep inside me and linger, infecting me with its odor. Necrosis. The stench of death. If I close my eyes, I can smell it today and it still makes my stomach turn and my heart plummet.

"OK, Sandra," I say. "You can cover up now."

She does. Her husband turns back toward us.

"Why didn't you do anything about this earlier, when you first felt a lump?" I ask as softly and as kindly as I can.

"I don't know." She looks down, guilt staining her face. "I know I should have. I'm just always so busy, taking care of everybody. We're raising my three grandchildren. My daughter, she's a sweet girl, but she's in and out of the house—she has drug problems—and my son-in-law is in prison. My husband, he works so hard on the farm, there's too much to do, and I have to help him there too. Me and him, we just never had the time to see a doctor. My family doctor—he's who I would've gone to—he passed away a couple years ago, so I don't really have a doctor. I didn't know who to call." She looks up, into my eyes, the fear visibly returning. "Do you think this is really serious? Please tell me it's not."

I don't know what to say. I know she has to be told how serious this is, but as an intern, it's not my place to do so. I reach to touch the back of her hand to comfort her.

Then, incredibly, as if he's been outside waiting, Dr. Weinberger charges in, relieving me of the need to answer the question, reminding me yet again that I'm a lowly intern. I'm a benchwarmer, watching the action from the sidelines, a doctor in name only.

Dr. Weinberger admits Sandra to the hospital. The next day she's brought to the operating room. Tentative diagnosis: breast cancer.

I try to convince myself that we can save Sandra, but a darkness envelops me as I scrub in. Today I'm a "second assistant," my two main tasks being (1) holding retractors and (2) watching.

Because the situation is so serious, Dr. Rabuchin, the attending general surgeon, has taken over Sandra's care and surgery. Dr. Weinberger will be his assistant. Of course, Weinberger wants Garth to scrub in instead of me, but Dr. Rabuchin vetoes him. After all, I was the first person to have contact with Sandra, and I know her case better than anybody.

As the surgery starts, it's still hard to look at all that decomposed, rotting flesh. We have smeared wintergreen inside our masks to help cover the smell, but the putrid odor overpowers everything. The OR now smells of death *and* wintergreen.

Using a massive scalpel, Dr. Rabuchin carefully removes the dead, necrotic tissue from the right side of Sandra's chest. As he gets rid of the slimy, stinking mush, it's clear that because Sandra waited so long to receive treatment, the breast has completely disintegrated.

Once Drs. Rabuchin and Weinberger are satisfied they've done everything they can with her chest, they remove a few lymph nodes. Then they call in Dr. Brandage, the plastic surgeon, to see what he can do to reconstruct and heal the area.

The place where Sandra's breast used to be is now a massive open wound, her underlying chest muscle exposed. Between her neck and her ribs, on the right side, she looks like someone who's been skinned alive.

At one point, I ask casually if I can stick around and assist Dr. Brandage. Predictably, Dr. Weinberger shoots me down. But Dr. Rabuchin overrides him and says I can stay. Weiney glares in my general direction as he leaves. I vow that when I get to be a resident, teaching interns, I will model Rabuchin and not Weinberger.

Dr. Brandage looks exactly what I think a young plastic surgeon should look like. Slender, fit, immaculate, with soft hands, smart eyes, and a cool, calm vibe. This guy owns the room without even trying. He asks me, "Have you ever done a skin graft?"

"No," I say, assuming I'll be shuttled off to the sidelines, as usual.

"Well," he says with a grin that's an invitation, "today's your lucky day, Doctor Youn."

Doctor Youn.

He emphasis the title, as if giving me both a boost and a reminder.

"I'd like to introduce you to the Dermatome."

He leads me over to the device we'll be using—metallic, with a hose like an industrial vacuum cleaner leading into a rectangular box, which contains the specialized blade. On the side, a knob presides over a bunch of numbers. The knob allows the doctor to control the thickness of the skin that's to be sliced off. The contraption looks like a meat slicer the Terminator would bring back from the future.

Dr. Brandage rubs his hands together and shakes out his fingers. "You know how delis have electric meatcutters so they can make their prosciutto super thin? That's kind of the idea here. Except instead of prosciutto, we're creating millimeter-thin slices of skin to make a graft."

He moves the Dermatome into position, just over Sandra's thigh. "You press the button to turn it on, then with very gentle downward pressure, go down her leg to harvest the skin."

I swallow. I almost say, "You sure you want me to do this?" but I catch myself and do as instructed. Within seconds, something comes over me—a feeling like a warm wave. I realize, simply, that this is one of the most awesome experiences of my life. It feels somehow...momentous.

In charge—feeling a sudden surge of pride and power—I gently press the Dermatome down onto Sandra's leg and watch it slice the upper layer of skin off her upper thigh. The layer is shockingly thin, looking like stretchy pink skin paper. I continue working the Dermatome until Dr. Brandage tells me I've removed enough skin. Soon, Sandra's thigh is covered with an adhesive plastic dressing that looks like cling wrap.

Dr. Brandage takes the skin graft and places it through a device that looks like a Play-Doh toy. "This is a mesher. By meshing the skin graft we can make it look like netting and that allows us to cover a much larger area and harvest less skin." He puts the skin graft into the mesher and lets me grind the crank. I feel like a kid again, cranking the handle of my Play-Doh noodle maker, as beautiful, symmetric tubes of pink Play-Doh smoothly flow out of the bottom.

Next, Dr. Brandage removes the graft and carefully spreads it over Sandra's open wound. He hands me the skin stapler and tells me to staple the edges of the graft into place. "We can't use sutures since they have a higher rate of infection, and with this wound, we have to avoid infection." He then begins to apply a bulky dressing onto the area, one layer at a time.

Performing this procedure excites and energizes me. Spending six months doing general surgery, I've felt lost, forgotten. *Where am I?* I've thought, and then even more pointedly—*Who am I?*

I answer my own questions.

I'm a plastic surgeon, I say to myself. *And working with Doctor Brandage, I'm* home.

We finish the procedure. We've cleaned out all the dead flesh. We've eliminated the stench. By those measures, you would call the surgery a success. But when the pathology report comes back, I don't see a victory. Sandra has invasive breast cancer. It has spread into her lymph nodes. The rest of the tests reveal extensive metastases in her bone, lungs, liver, and brain.

All we can do is send her home to die.

* * *

I visit Sandra the day she checks out of the hospital. I pause at the doorway before I enter her room. She sits in a chair next to the hospital bed. She no longer wears an expression of deep fear. Instead she looks lost.

And sad. Terribly sad.

I walk into the room, not sure what I will say, how to comfort her. She smiles when I approach her. I smile back.

"Looking forward to getting back home?" I ask. "Bet it'll be nice to go to church on Sunday, won't it?"

Sandra's face lights up. "Oh, yeah, it'll sure be nice to be home. And get back to church." She smiles again, bashfully. "I love to sing. I just wish I had a better voice." She chuckles a little. I chuckle with her. "And I can't wait to see my grandkids. I hear they're baking me a cake. Oh, the mess them kids make! And guess who's gonna have to clean it up?"

Now she laughs out loud. I laugh along with her—until I imagine her, full of cancer, even now cleaning up after everyone.

"I'm going to give you my number," I say. "If there's anything you need, if there's anything I can do, please let me know."

I jot down my cell phone number on the back of my card and hand it to her.

"Thank you, Doctor Youn. That is so nice. But I'd expect nothing less from a young man from Greenville." She takes the card and rubs her finger along the edge as if it's a check for $100,000.

"You know, you might want to consider talking with somebody about your feelings, about the diagnosis. This is about the hardest thing a person can go through. Sometimes it's easier to talk to a therapist or a minister than it is to your family."

"That's real kind of you, Doctor Youn. Truth is, it's not me I'm worried about. It's my grandkids. Who's gonna look after them? I don't want them to walk down the wrong path. I don't want them to make the same mistakes their mom made. The mistakes *I* made."

Her eyes begin to well up with tears.

"And my husband...he's lost without me. I get so upset thinking about what's gonna happen to him." Sandra turns away from me and gazes out the window. Tears stream down her cheeks. "Who's gonna look after him? I just can't help thinking, if I'd took care of myself as good as I took care of them, maybe we wouldn't be in this mess. What's my husband going to do without me?" She lowers her head and weeps quietly.

I don't know what to say. I have no words. I reach over and silently hold her hand. After several seconds, she wipes her face with a tissue and looks back out the window.

"Live and learn, right?" she says.

"Yes," I say. "Live and learn."

I never hear from Sandra again.

She dies two months later.

Twenty years later, she still shows up in my dreams.

3

Wasting Away Again in Grand Haven

Eyes closed, head thrown back, I punish the strings of my old black Telecaster and belt out the chorus to "Margaritaville."

Oh, yeah!

I own this song.

I own this stage.

I own this entire *room*.

OK, it's my living room I own, and it's Saturday morning and I'm singing and playing along to Jimmy Buffett's *Songs You Know by Heart* on my CD player. But still.

* * *

March–April.

Residency, year one.

My social life, such as it is, consists of catching a few half-awake hours here and there with Amy. I rarely see the interns from my group anymore, except in passing in the hallway or catching a quick, groggy snack break. I don't have friends, as such. My close friends from med school have scattered all over the country. Amy, as usual, cuts to the chase.

"You have no life," she says one day as I try to focus on some movie on TV while keeping my eyelids from crashing down over my exhausted pupils. "All you do is work and sleep. You need to get out more. Expand your horizons."

"I hear you. One question. What are you talking about?"

"I don't know. Maybe take up a hobby."

"A hobby? You mean like drawing my own comic books or dressing up and doing role-playing at *Star Trek* conventions?"

"Uh, no. Let's think about this." Amy scrunches her face in that cute way she has when she's solving a complex, challenging problem. "OK, we know what you want to be when you grow up. A plastic surgeon. But when that happens you're going to be under a lot of pressure, right?"

"No! Pressure? I can't imagine that!"

"Whatever. So, you need a release. Something where you can blow off steam. OK, just for fun, let's say this doctor thing doesn't work out."

"For *fun*?"

"Work with me. You crash, you burn, you drop out of residency. What would be your second choice?"

"Easy. I'd like to be Jimmy Buffett."

"Great. And your third choice? Because I'm pretty sure your second choice is already taken...by *Jimmy freaking Buffett.*"

"I know. I'm thinking of joining a Jimmy Buffett cover band."

"Because you look so much like Jimmy Buffett?"

"Exactly!"

"I'm being serious."

"Me too."

"Really?" A pause. She's trying to reconcile the image of a dutiful surgeon with that of an inebriated Parrot Head. Scanning my face for signs I'm putting her on, backing off, buying it, stating a fact. "You're not kidding around."

"I've actually been checking out bulletin boards in music stores, seeing if anybody's looking for a rhythm guitarist who knows the entire Jimmy Buffett catalog by heart."

"Which would be you?"

"Which would be me."

"I find that...how shall I put this...somewhat"—Amy looks up at the ceiling grappling for a particular word, nods, finds it—"disturbing."

"I know. Awesome, right?" I say. "Hey, I'll need a roadie. Someone I can trust to handle my cable. And a groupie of course."

Amy raises her hand. "I'd like to apply for both jobs."

"You're hired."

"That's it? That's the entire interview?"

"There's a more extensive vetting process later. I think you'll do fine. Well, it's a short list. You're the only applicant."

She snuggles into my shoulder. "Better be."

* * *

For the next couple of weeks, I scour the bulletin boards at the local music stores in search of Jimmy Buffett cover bands that need a rhythm guitarist who can sing. Nothing. No sign of needy Parrot Head musicians anywhere. I go to plan B. The internet. I find a local Parrot Head club website and shoot off an email to the general Parrot Head population. Within days, I receive a reply. The webmaster, a guy named Duke, has in fact been considering forming a Jimmy Buffett cover band. *Great minds,* I think. Duke says that once summer starts, there will be no shortage of gigs at bars, beach clubs, and Parrot Head club meetings.

I email back: "Duke, hey! Tony here. I'd love to be in your band. I play rhythm guitar and I sing. Full disclosure. I'm a mediocre guitarist and a mediocre singer. But I'm really interested and if you don't find anyone else, I'll audition for you. Plus, I have my own gear! And my own roadie!"

Duke replies within ten minutes.

"Wow! You really know how to sell yourself! You're in! We just need a percussionist and we've got a band!"

A week later, Duke emails me again.

"Found a guy! Name's Troy. Lots of experience. Drums, congas, very Jimmy! Our first rehearsal is Saturday at noon, my house! We're gonna party with a purpose!"

Wow. Could it be true? Am I going to be a surgeon *and* a rock star?

* * *

We meet in Duke's finished basement, dimly lit, his walls plastered with maps of Florida and Parrot Head posters and allegedly soundproofed to protect his wife and young son from losing their hearing, and Duke from getting divorced. Duke is a few years older than I am, early thirties. But Troy, the new recruit drummer, is nearly bald, a few lonely neon silver hairs poking up from the top of his scalp, and he sports a straggly gray mustache and beard. His flabby stomach flops over his belt and pops out beneath his oversize Hawaiian shirt. Troy admits to turning fifty-eight on his last birthday. He seems to know every Jimmy Buffett song ever recorded and despite an occasional confused, wan look that reminds me of someone in the middle of a three-day cleanse, he is pleasant and highly enthusiastic. Duke immediately surprises me with strong guitar skills and a sweet melodic voice, while Troy keeps perfect time. Winding up our rehearsal after a couple of hours, I think this could actually work. I am already on the road to becoming a rock legend. Or at least a guitar player in a semidecent Jimmy Buffett cover band.

"Well," Duke says, nodding, grinning, "that was pretty awesome."

"Totally," Troy says.

"I love your voice," I tell Duke.

"Totally," Troy says.

"Thanks," Duke says. "Oh, listen, one thing you guys should know. I don't talk."

"Huh?" I say.

"At gigs. I freeze. I can play, I can sing, I can even dance, but I don't talk."

"I don't talk either," Troy says. "Kills my image."

"What image?" I say.

"The rock star sex thing. Strong. Silent. Groupies love that."

"You said you were married," I say.

"I am," Troy says, winking. "In Muskegon."

We stare at him.

"You know what they say," Troy continues, "'what happens in Grand Haven stays in Grand Haven.'"

He winks again for emphasis. I look at Duke, like *WTF?*

Duke shrugs. "I don't judge. Anyway, about the talking. I clam up. Got nothing to say. I turn into a mime." He raises his hands, stuck in an invisible box.

"I'll talk," I say, imagining myself all debonair and witty, wooing massive crowds of Parrot Heads from East Lansing to Detroit. "I'll intro the songs, whatever."

"Great," Duke says.

"We need a name," Troy says.

We all nod dumbly and then for the next few minutes we toss out idiotic possibilities, each somehow worse than the next. Finally, someone suggests Migration, the name of a Jimmy Buffett song. It sticks.

"Migration," I say.

"I love it," Duke says.

"Totally," Troy says.

Thus, our band is born.

* * *

We rehearse when we can in Duke's basement. We play open mics in redneck bars in the middle of nowhere, often before audiences of seven people, two being Duke's wife and Amy. Troy's wife never shows. He rarely talks about her except to complain that she's always held him back, squashing his lifelong dream to become what he was born to be: a rock 'n' roll drummer. I'm no shrink but based on how Troy hits on every available (or unavailable for that matter) woman in the immediate area and the posse of twenty-somethings he seems to hang out with, I think it's safe to say he's in the middle of a midlife crisis.

As spring rolls around and the weather turns balmy, we book our first real—although still unpaid—gig: a Parrot Head club party in front of 150 people. We roar through our set list, each song earning more applause than the last. I can't believe it. We're actually sort of good. Or at least not horrible. Standing onstage after winding up our version of "Volcano," I feel a bolt of energy and excitement crackling through me. As Duke tunes up and Troy wipes his sweat-soaked brow, I grab the mic and ad-lib, "How you all doing?"

A roar from the crowd.

Feeling giddy, I press on. "Awright!!! You having fun?"

Even bigger roar from the crowd.

I whirl toward Duke. "How you doing, Duke?"

"Me?" For just a moment he looks like the most un–rock star musician ever to take a stage. "Oh...I'm...fine."

Another roar from the crowd.

"Hey, everyone, what do you think about our lead singer, Duke?"

Monster roar from the crowd as Duke waves sheepishly and then counts us down into the next song.

By the time we finish our set, I'm flying. I'm Jackson Browne, Tom Petty, Zac Brown. Hell, I'm Jimmy Buffett!

Inebriated men and women swarm the stage, slap hands with me. Someone hands me a beer. Behind me Troy laughs and flirts with two women in bikinis who look like they could still be in college. Duke, meanwhile, talks intently with a gray-haired guy in a ponytail. I decide right then to grow my hair out. Shortly after this party, we book another gig at an outdoor tiki bar. Then another gig at a private beach club. Then another and another. Then the incredible happens.

Migration starts making money.

* * *

Summer hits and we're hotter than the weather, playing two or three gigs per weekend. Somehow I manage to juggle my two worlds. Wearing my long white coat, slipping my stethoscope over my head, playing doctor and saving humankind in all three Grand Rapids hospitals. And wearing my loose-fitting, loud Hawaiian shirt, slipping my Telecaster over my head, and playing "Margaritaville" in Grand Haven, Michigan. I go from little sleep to almost no sleep, running on fumes, but I don't mind. I have a secret identity. I'm a superhero, and my power is creating tropical rock party tunes. I'm a double threat. A high-powered hyphenate. I'm a doctor–rock star.

Thankfully, whenever my ego threatens to inflate, Amy lovingly brings me crashing back to earth. "Honey, not to split hairs, but you're actually a first-year resident and a rhythm guitar player and backup singer in a local Jimmy Buffett *cover* band, but fine, live the dream, baby."

One Friday night we book a gig in Saugatuck, a tiny beach town an hour away on the Kalamazoo River, known for its abundance of art galleries, tourists, and sweeping, undulating sand dunes. I check my schedule and realize that I will be coming off an all-nighter, a thirty-six-hour shift. *What I do to entertain*, I tell myself in the mirror, loading up my recently grown-out hair with a fistful of gel. Digging my new rock star look, I stuff some clothes into my overnight bag so I can hit the road once my shift is over.

Bleary-eyed, putting out fires all night, not finding a moment to catch my breath, not catching five minutes of sleep, I stagger into my apartment at six p.m., grab my bag, and swing by to pick up my roadie/groupie, Amy. Yes, Amy has embraced Migration almost as much as I have, and, truthfully, I need her. Without her, I might find myself halfway to Saugatuck before I realized I'd forgotten my guitar. Or my head, for that matter. Before we leave, Amy goes over the checklist in her head, makes sure I've got speakers, amps, microphones, cables, my tropical shirt, and my mojo. Then we head out.

We meet Duke and Troy at the gig, a bar on the beach lined with tiki torches. As we set up, guests arrive, fifty or sixty in all, many in Tommy Bahama shirts and grass skirts, a few wearing actual parrot heads. We start playing and as we go into "Changes in Latitudes, Changes in Attitudes," I feel a tingle of goose bumps. We've never sounded tighter. Troy's drumming feels like a perfect, thumping pulse. Duke's acoustic guitar twanging gets to the heart of each song and his voice covers every lyric with an idyllic, tropical island sweetness. We finish our set and the crowd—wasted away, wild, ecstatic—not only goes nuts, but they won't let us leave. They insist on an encore. We stumble around on stage trying to settle on a song when someone in the crowd shouts, "We'll pay you ten dollars if you play 'Margaritaville'!"

We play "Margaritaville."

Then someone else screams, "Ten more for 'Southern Cross'!"

We play "Southern Cross."

And then "Son of a Son of a Sailor" and "Pencil Thin Mustache" and "Brown-Eyed Girl" and five more encores until Duke loses his voice, Troy's fingers go numb, and I'm so tired my hair falls asleep. Duke waves his handkerchief in surrender. We take our final bows to screaming and applauding, feeling exhausted and exhilarated.

Blind drunk on the adulation I've yet to receive from popping cysts and stripping veins at my day job, I drop my head onto my Telecaster and seriously start to weigh my career choice.

"Come on, Bono, let's pack this stuff up." Amy whacks me on the side of the head, snapping me out of my trance.

"Some gig," I mumble.

"Yep. Probably your best. Unplug that wire, will you?"

Ten minutes later, the bar's jukebox blaring behind us, the party still raging, Duke lost, and Troy chasing coed tail, Amy and I pack everything into the car. As I slide my guitar into the RAV4's way back, I catch a smile curling on her face.

"What?" I say.

"Don't let this go to your head," she says, lightly kissing me. "You're pretty great, *Doctor* Youn."

"You too," I say.

"Now, let's go home. And hand over the keys. I'm driving."

"Good call." I fish through my pockets for the keys.

Suddenly, a tricked-out, oversized van with Bacardi Rum decals plastered all along its side rumbles into the parking lot and screeches to a stop. The side panel slides open and three long-haired, long-limbed young women wearing bikinis so skimpy they look like they're made out of dental floss teeter out on towering stiletto heels, giggling, swaying, and sashaying toward the bar. I freeze in midkey search.

"Wow, unbelievable," I say. "Those are the actual Bacardi girls. Live. At our gig. *Live*. And pretty much fully naked. Very nice of them to come. Very thoughtful. Maybe we should buy them a drink, you know, just to be polite...."

I feel Amy's laser stare hot enough to bore a hole right through my forehead. "Focus. Eyes front."

"Yes." I resume patting myself down. "Keys."

A roar rippling from inside causes us to turn toward the bar and try to get a glimpse inside.

"They're in the bag," I say.

"You're not kidding," Amy says. "Completely hammered."

"I'm talking about the keys," I say.

She rolls her eyes and now we laugh as I open the car, unzip the overnight bag, and start a new search.

A thunderous roar, followed by a wave of howling, cheering, and clapping, comes from inside the bar. I shoot Amy my irresistible puppy dog face.

"Fine," she says, rolling her gorgeous eyes and shaking her head. "Let's check it out."

Side by side, we edge into the bar looking for an opening that we might squeeze through. A crowd has formed a horseshoe around the bar's one pool table. People are whistling, clapping, laughing. Duke stands off to the side, his mouth open wide in what appears to be equal parts amazement and horror. I steer Amy toward him. Somehow we manage to zigzag through bystanders and arrive at his side, creating an opening where we manage to get a clear, unobstructed view of the pool table. A Bacardi girl lies across the green felt. Troy, the bearded, balding, midlife-crisising sex machine, bends over her, slurping a shot of rum out of her navel.

"Wow," Amy says.

"Double wow," Duke says. He nods at a woman in her fifties standing a few feet away, her arms clasped tight across her chest. She doesn't look happy. In fact, not even sunglasses can hide the fact that she looks as far from happy as a woman can look.

"No," I say. "That can't be."

"It is," Duke says.

"Well, the good news is," I say, "Troy's wife finally came to a gig."

"The bad news is," Amy says, "Troy's wife finally came to a gig."

I look back at the pool table. Troy pours another shot of rum into the Bacardi girl's navel, bends over, and, to window-shattering cheering, slurps, stands, and raises both arms in triumph, rum dripping from his gray beard. When I turn to see Troy's wife's reaction, she is gone, baby, gone.

Amy and I return to Grand Rapids. I sleep most of the ride back, crawl into bed in my apartment, and conk out for eight blissful hours.

That night I receive an email from Duke.

Troy has left the band for personal reasons.

Migration is now a duo.

* * *

One day in June, after plowing through one eighty-hour week after another, I start to imagine a dim thimble of light appearing in a distant tunnel, signifying the end of my first year of residency.

In a month or so, I will no longer be an intern.

I will discard that title and become a resident.

It seems like both years ago and yesterday that I walked through the halls of the hospital for the first time wearing my long white coat with "Anthony Youn, M.D." stitched above the pocket. That day a nurse called me "Doctor Youn." Confused, I whirled around, thinking, *Is my dad here?*

Now, self-proclaimed vein stripping virtuoso, adept at catheter insertion, the go-to escort to the radiology department, and with more pilonidal cyst excisions than I care to count, I feel not only more confident, but I feel at home. As my last days of being an intern come to a close, I accept an invitation to dinner at my parents' house. Running late, I have no time to change and walk into the living room wearing my long white coat. My dad, reading a Korean newspaper, sitting in his favorite chair facing the window, snaps the paper closed and stands to greet me. He takes one step and stops. He stares at me, a strange expression appearing on his face that I can't quite identify.

"Anthony Youn, M.D." He stares at my name above my pocket. He comes over to me and tentatively rubs his hand over my name. He smiles shyly.

"Now another Doctor Youn in the family," he says.

"Yeah." I watch my father continue to trace my name with his fingers. Behind us, my mother stands in the doorway. I can feel her smile without even looking at her.

"Maybe take a picture," my dad says and my mother heads out of the living room, returning with a camera.

"Stand together," my mother says.

My dad and I put our arms around each other's shoulders and smile into the camera.

"You're gonna be world famous plastic surgeon," my dad says. "You may not be world famous cardiothoracic surgeon or neurosurgeon or even colorectal surgeon but that's OK."

"Say cheese," my mother says.

"Cheese," my father and I say simultaneously.

"Good job," my dad says, moving his hand from my name gently to my cheek.

Watching him, I finally identify the expression I saw on his face earlier, a look that has remained fastened in my mind's eye since that moment.

The look I saw was pride.

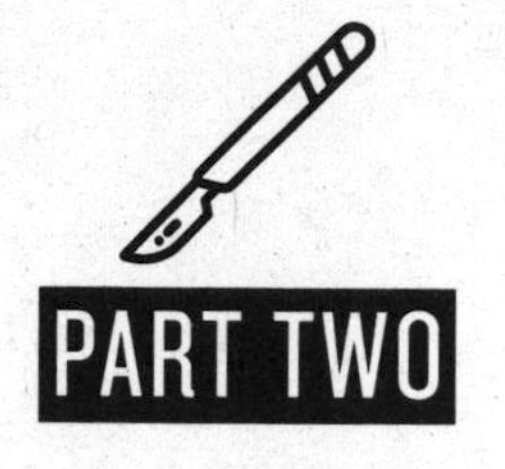

PART TWO

RESIDENCY—YEAR TWO

4

Don't Get Sick in July

Take it from me. Don't get sick in July.

In the medical world, we refer to treating patients from July 1–31 as the July Effect. That's the month when hospitals are teeming with first- and second-year residents who don't know shit.

Who has two thumbs and doesn't know shit? *This guy.*

* * *

Residency—year two.

July 2.

One day after second-year orientation.

Literally, my first night on call as a resident.

I'm no longer an intern.

I am a big bad resident working trauma surgery.

This is my hospital now.

I am in charge.

For what I hope will be better. And pray not be for worse.

I have been assigned my own intern, an unfortunate clueless scut monkey named Tariq, who clings to me like my shadow.

After today he will arrive an hour ahead of me and perform all the crap duties and fill out all the soul-sucking paperwork my residents stuck me with last year when I was an unfortunate, clueless, scut monkey intern. Tariq, as eager as I was, a mini me, loves it, lives for it, eats it all up like ice cream.

The truth is I'm a pushover. I like Tariq, even though I've known him less than a day. And unlike many residents I know who treat interns like personal valets, butlers, or, in some cases, indentured servants, I consider Tariq my wingman, my running partner. Completing medical school in his native Pakistan, Tariq is a little tentative, sort of quiet, and extremely nervous. He also struggles with English. So far, we've had more luck communicating with extreme facial expressions and international nonverbal hand signals than with conversation.

Ten p.m. I need a pick-me-up. We plunder a vending machine for soft drinks with the most caffeine, snap them open in unison, chug them like we're at a sleep-deprived, antiseptic frat party, squash the cans, lob them into the recycling bin, and shuffle down a hallway lit by horror film lighting, the only sound the intermittent creepy beeping of a distant heart monitor. A few feet in front of us a nurse bursts out of a patient's room.

"Call a code!" she yells to the receptionist sitting at the nurse's station, then she looks in my direction. "My patient's coding! I need you to run this code! You're a resident, right?"

I look left, right, and behind me.

I look at Tariq who shrugs and mouths, *No English*.

Gulp.

She's talking to *me*.

Is it too late to hide in a closet?

"Let's go," I say, hoping she hasn't noticed that my voice sounded like Elmo from *Sesame Street* after sucking on helium.

I run after the nurse into the room, Tariq so close behind he's practically inside my white coat. The patient, a woman in her seventies, lies like a corpse in her hospital bed. Her face has gone pale as an albino ghost. Her breathing, intermittent, slow, and raspy, revs once and then stops. I don't know much, but I have seen enough to know that she is about to die. Right now, my job—my only job—is to stop her from dying.

Panic grips me. *Holy crap, I don't remember my advanced lifesaving!*

Our second-year orientation included a course in Advanced Cardiac Life Support (ACLS), but I have not spent a minute reviewing the manual. I intended to go over it before I started my second year, I really did, but being in a Jimmy Buffett cover band got in the way. You have to have your priorities straight. Bottom line, I'm not feeling all that confident about running this code.

"What do we do?"

The nurse.

Looking at me, imploring me, her eyes wide as quarters.

"Well," I say, now searching Tariq's face for a clue. He stares back at me; his panic is a mirror of mine. "We really should"—I pause and then scream as if we're in the middle of a huge crowd—*"start CPR and hook her up to a cardiac monitor!"*

To this day I have no idea why I shout this. But it does get everyone moving. Fast. One nurse starts chest compressions while another nurse exits briefly and returns rolling in a boxy monitor on a stand. She scrambles to untangle a bunch of wires, and then the two of them start hooking up the patient. Feeling like a statue of a completely ineffectual doctor, I look again at Tariq for...what? I'm not sure. Help? Guidance? An answer? More sugar and caffeine?

"Ventricular fibrillation," he whispers, tilting his head toward the heart monitor. I follow his eyes and on the monitor I see that the patient is indeed in ventricular fibrillation.

This is the heart rhythm that immediately precedes death.

The first nurse resumes chest compressions while the second nurse starts running medications into an IV.

I lead Tariq to a corner of the room and turn my back to the nurses so they can't hear what an idiot I am.

"Do you know what to do?" I ask him.

He shrugs, either having no idea or not understanding. I try a couple of feeble hand gestures. I thump my heart and then drop my head onto my chest to indicate a dead person. He blinks at me, desperately trying to crack my code, to catch on, as if he's been recruited to play in the life-and-death version of Charades.

I dangle my hands at my side and shake my wrists.

I close my eyes.

My mind goes dark.

Nothing.

Think, Tony, think.

"Review book!" I scream in a stage whisper.

Tariq looks at me, lost.

I reach my hand into his pocket and pull out his mini ACLS manual.

"Ventricular fibrillation!" he shouts, startling the nurses.

"That's it, absolutely!" I announce to the nurses. I then whisper to Tariq, "I'm pretty sure."

Tariq nods furiously, snatches back the manual and rifles through it. He stops at a page and reads frantically, using his finger to guide him. He stabs the page with his finger and looks up. Tariq slaps his hands together violently and makes a buzzing sound.

"Tariq, this is no time for mime. What does it say?"

"You need...*shock*," he says.

"You're right!" I stride toward the patient, stop, put myself in reverse, back up to Tariq. "What setting?"

"One hundred twenty joules," Tariq says, reading, his eyes riveted to the book.

"You sure?"

Tariq follows his finger across the page, nods even more violently. "Yes. Absolute. One hundred twenty joules."

"Defibrillation," I say, returning to the nurses. They look stunned. And then I say as dramatically as a Broadway actor, "Get me the paddles!"

The first nurse rummages beneath the monitor, shoves the paddles into my hands.

"One hundred twenty joules!"

The nurse adjusts the power setting.

"Clear!" I yell, channeling Dr. McDreamy from *Grey's Anatomy*.

I place the paddles on the patient's chest.

"STOP!" the nurse screams.

I yank the paddles off the patient and hold them in midair above her chest. The nurse grabs my hands and moves the paddles to a different spot on the patient's body.

One more second and I would have shocked her liver.

"Clear!" I yell again, softer, my voice starting to wobble. I press the defibrillation button.

The patient jerks slightly and for an instant the heart monitor goes wild. Then it completely stops. The nurses, Tariq, and I stand side by side in a line like backup singers waiting for the chorus, staring at the monitor for what seems like minutes, praying she gets a new cardiac rhythm.

Beep...beep...beep.

Normal sinus rhythm.

She's saved.

We saved her.

I whistle out a breath of relief.

Within seconds, two internal medicine residents enter the room and take over for me. I step aside and nod to them as cool as James Dean, but feeling as if I'm about to faint. I slip out of the room, Tariq by my side.

"Putting out fires," I say.

He nods and chuckles. He has no idea what I'm talking about.

An hour later Tariq has turned in for the night and I stagger into the call room. I'd promised myself earlier that I would try to get at least some sleep. But I abandon that idea. All I can see in my mind's eye is me shocking that poor woman's liver. *Thank God that nurse moved my hands....*

I fish my dog-eared ACLS manual out of my overnight bag.

I study it cover-to-cover until dawn.

* * *

Trauma.

An injury or wound to living tissue requiring surgery.

Them.

* * *

On any given night, I treat extreme life-threatening injuries and wounds caused by gunshots, stabbings, bar fights, animal bites, car accidents, workplace incidents, and occasional acts of God. I try to detach myself and focus on my job, on my doctoring, on my surgical skills and training, assisting attending doctors in any way I am needed.

I succeed.

Mostly.

* * *

Trauma.

A disordered psychic or behavioral state resulting from mental or emotional stress.

Me.

* * *

One night.

Five trauma codes.

Ambulances stacked up. ER packed. People roaming, waiting, praying. Patients in distress, in pain, on edge. Smells swirl, hints of antiseptic cream, disinfectant, fear, and death. We put out one fire, another flares. We fight to save lives. We win some. We lose others. Two patients die.

On these nights, when all hell breaks loose, the staff notices which residents are on call. If horrible nights in the ER seem to occur when the same resident is on call, the staff refers to that resident as a "black cloud." I have been known for my sunny disposition. But during my second consecutive night of hell in the ER, I notice the receptionist at the nursing station looking at me as if I'm a cumulonimbus.

"It's not me," I tell her. "I am not a black cloud. Think how insane it would be if I *wasn't* on call."

She laughs. I buy some time. I'm not yet a black cloud.

But the year is yet young.

* * *

I try to preserve my strength.

I attempt to feed my spirit.

The key is sleep.

I can make it on one hour.

I call two a premium.

Three, a gift.

When the action in the ER lulls, I slink into the call room to regroup and recharge. The call room is the size of a freshman-year dorm room and decorated with the charm of the Bates Motel. A single bed. A hunchbacked mattress. Sandpaper polyester sheets. A twenty-three-thread-count air-thin blanket apparently stitched together from a bunch of used burlap bags and guaranteed to make your private parts chafe. A vinyl pillow that seems to have been dipped in someone's hair gel. At least I hope it's hair gel. No window. A physically challenged desk chair from Big Lots missing one wheel. A rickety desk leaning like a drop-dead drunk into the wall with a telephone, the first Dell desktop ever made, a cranky television set where everyone's face is a shade of alien green, and a portable table fan that howls like a chainsaw massacre when you turn it on. Above the desk a bookshelf with a few medical books and a Bible. Just in case. Stained industrial carpet that should be euthanized. Three pictures in dusty faux wood frames above the bed, one depicting sailboats and a seashore, one a bowl of fruit, one something either vaguely religious or strangely erotic, depending on just how tired you are.

The call room hugs the wall around the corner from the patient rooms and on the other side shares a wall with the elevator. Every twenty seconds the elevator door opens, arriving with a piercing *ding* that echoes through your skull like an air raid siren. And the call room *smells*, a stomach-flipping mix of flop sweat, body odor, ammonia, decomposing magazines, and medical failure.

One reckless night, inspired from scenes of doctors on TV soaps who sneak into the call room to hook up during quiet moments between treating gunshot victims, Amy and I decide to christen the call room ourselves. We lock the door and get as far as a nervous kiss when the elevator's constant dinging and the stanky stench of moldy *Cosmos* doesn't just kill but executes the mood.

"What *is* that?" Amy's face folds into a nose-wrinkling frown.

"You mean the elevator? Or the smell?"

"Yes," Amy says.

"Call rooms are much nicer on *General Hospital*," I say. "But that's TV. This is real."

"Really real. Disgustingly real. Buzz-killing real."

Being a sensitive male, I whisper into her ear before burying my face in her neck, trying desperately to recapture the vibe and return to the intimacy. Guys will do anything for even the remote *possibility* of action. "Ignore that stuff. Shut your eyes, close your ears, and take in the scent of my manliness."

She explodes with laughter before nearly tumbling off the bed.

"All right," I say. "I know this is not ideal. I get that. I'm totally sensitive to how you feel. I always want you to be comfortable. So let's just have a quickie and get the hell out of here."

My pager *beeps*.

"And that concludes tonight's very special episode of *Love on Call,*" Amy says and chuckles.

* * *

I know myself. I'm slightly obsessive. I thrive on structure and routine. The opposite of life on call when anything, or nothing, can happen. Each shift is fluid, varying hour to hour from eerily quiet to the wild, wild west. I rarely see my group from first year anymore, but when I do, I ask them how they approach their nights on call and try to learn from them. Jessica seems almost afraid to fall asleep. She wants to keep alert. Fall asleep and you run the risk of sleep drunkenness, awakening in a delirious state. Shelley, the gunner, busies herself by studying. Yes, *studying*. *Sleep-deprived* studying. As residents, we're still technically students with thousands of pages of medical literature to absorb. Jessica reads and knits, and Garth—well, Garth, I believe, is from another planet where the advanced life forms do not require sleep—is always raring to go, and perpetually, maddeningly, freakingly *perky.*

Conrad approaches his nights on call like a character trapped in the latest *American Pie* sequel. He knows he should study and at least try to get some sleep. But he's either so zoned out that he watches hour after hour of TV in a comatose state, or he's so horny that he flirts shamelessly and endlessly with the nurses. Life for him, with everyone in scrubs, is like one big adult pajama party, interrupted with episodes of blood and pus.

I am committed to getting my work done and grabbing as much sleep as I can. I round on my patients right after dinner, making sure everyone is "tucked in for the night." Translation: Tariq the intern has checked their vitals and gone over their labs and I've checked and double-checked Tariq. Then I knock out an hour or so of trying to stop my eyes from crossing as I study, hit my pillow hard, sack out, and saw as many logs as I can. And I am talking about *my* pillow. I've brought my own comfy cozy pillow from home, the real secret to tricking myself into believing I'm actually snuggling into the sacred space of my own bed. Bringing my own pillow was actually Amy's brilliant idea and it works surprisingly well. Soon as I hit the lights and find the cool side of the pillow, *my* pillow, I conk out like a stressed narcoleptic. I consider sneaking my teddy bear into the call room too, but I'm afraid of damaging my Dr. Bad Boy resident image. Hey, a man can dream.

My sleep system is nearly flawless, almost fail-proof, providing me with at least two hours of shut-eye a night, often more.

That's *nearly* flawless and *almost* fail-proof. There is one minor flaw. Small thing. Not a major problem.

I'm addicted to eBay.

I freaking love it.

I love the hunt, the chase, the competition.

OK, I'm lying.

I love to win.

That's what it's all about.

Winning.

Winning, though, costs money, more money than I should spend, more money than I actually *have*.

At least I'm not wasting my money on a bunch of frivolous crap. That's what I keep telling my delusional mind anyway.

Because I buy comic books.

Classics.

I go after only vintage stuff such as...

The Avengers: issue number four. First edition. Issue date March 1, 1964. Very fine condition.

It's dead at the nurses' station. I sit down at the computer. The computer in the call room is a worthless piece of crap, and besides, I don't want to go on eBay alone in the call room. That feels sad, pathetic, dirty. I'm not ashamed relaxing publicly with this harmless distraction, outbidding and outsmarting a bunch of creepy lowlifes for what only I know to be a classic comic, an overlooked treasure, a gem, an *investment.* I don't care if the nurses know what I'm doing. Hell, I'm not looking at porn, like Conrad.

I log onto eBay, scroll through the comics, and stop, stunned. I can't believe what I see on the page in front of me. *Avengers,* first edition. Issue number four, opening bid $200.

Are you kidding me?

I know this comic to be worth at least twice that much.

I bid $200.

I feel cocky. Bunch of losers in some hovel of an apartment or a fifty-year-old sad sack living in his parent's basement going up against me, having no idea that I'm a freaking *doctor*. Piece of cake.

Somebody bids $220.

"What? You bastard."

I say this aloud.

Too loud.

A nurse doing paperwork a few desks away fidgets, adjusts her glasses, tries not to glance in the direction of the guy swearing at the computer.

I wait a few more seconds and then up my bid to $240.

Ping.

The lowlife clown overbids me, goes to $260.

I grunt.

Yeah, jerkoff, I know your game. I'm a doctor, dumbass. I make $1,000 a week. Hey, Mr. Loser, in your two-hundred-square-foot mobile home. Take that.

I type in $300.

Then $310 hits me like a slap.

"*Whaaaaaaaaat?*"

The word slips out, stretching about five syllables. The nurse doing paperwork clears her throat. Translation: Please stop acting like a freak before I report you to HR.

"Sorry," I say. "I'm just writing up a report...."

She laughs, covers her mouth quickly with her fist and a fake cough.

I casually type in $320, check the time ticking away. We've got less than a minute left before the bids close.

I wait.

Nothing.

OK, I've got him. Too rich for his blood. And I'd call $320—while a little extravagant, a little nuts, hell, we're talking almost a third of my weekly salary—a totally reasonable price. I mean come on, it's *The Avengers. Issue number four, from March 1, 1964!*

Ping.

He's back.

At $340.

Forty-six seconds and counting. I stand up, point at the screen, and say, reading his screen name, "Who the hell are you, Silver Surfer Voodoo Man? What kind of a stupid screen name is that?"

"Doctor Youn, are you all right?"

The nurse.

She removes her glasses and looks at me with genuine concern.

"Oh, no, no, no, yeah, I'm fine, great, just doing some...research, ha-ha ha, yeah, no, great, no worries, I'm *fine.*"

Try to regroup. I smile at her like a lunatic, yank off my glasses, and massage the bridge of my nose. The nurse dips her head and returns to her work. But I can see she's looking at me out of the corner of her eye, ready to make a break for it when I finally snap.

I shove my glasses back on and stare at the computer screen, hard.

Twenty-eight seconds left.

Silver Surfer Voodoo Man, my ass. What a childish screen name. Look at my screen name, loser. I am Doctor freaking Doom!!!

I type in $350.

He types in $360.

I type in $370.

He types in $380.

Twenty seconds to go.

My heart thumps in my chest like I'm in supraventricular tachycardia.

I pound the keys, type in $400.

Fifteen seconds.

He types in $420.

I growl like a beast hungry to feed.

Sweat pours down my forehead.

Ten seconds.

"You will not defeat..."

Five seconds.

I type in $450.

"*...Doctor Doom!*"

The auction closes.

"*Yeah, baby! In your face, Silver Surfer Voodoo fool! I win!!!*"

I leap to my feet, raise both hands, lean over to the nurse, and high-five her.

"Congratulations," she says, high-fiving me back with a weird combination of worry and pity, having no idea what just happened.

Drained, wasted, but triumphant, I melt into my chair. I do some quick math. Then I remember I have to pay the piper. I calculate that in less than ten minutes I have spent 45 percent of my weekly paycheck, before taxes, on a comic book.

But I *won*.

I freaking *won*!

Now I just have to explain to Amy that I'll be eating Ramen noodles for the foreseeable future.

5

The Decisions You Make

1:47 a.m.

Drunk, furious, his world catapulting at him in fractured frames of pulsing scarlet, his sightline whirling, the young man stumbles out of his small house, squeezes behind the wheel of his car. Ignoring his seat belt, he screeches down his driveway at thirty miles an hour. He swerves for no reason, slams into a parked car, swears, backs up, straightens the wheels, and veers onto a main street. He runs a red light, cuts off one car, sideswipes another, and rams a van in the right lane. The car jumps the curb and plows into a mailbox. The young man's head snaps back. His field of vision clouds. He feels a warm liquid dribbling down his forehead. He drops his chin onto the steering wheel and exhales, his breath fogging the windshield. He hears voices. He lifts his head and the voices become rumbles. They morph into shouting. He peers ahead and squints into a sea of throbbing blue light. He stomps on the floor of the car with his frayed and cracked cowboy boot, searching for the accelerator. His boot nicks the gas pedal and falls off. He curses, moans, and two police officers whip open the car door, haul him outside, his legs dragging on the pavement. One cop presses a cloth onto the young man's forehead, which in seconds becomes sopped with blood. The other cop stuffs him into the back seat of their cruiser.

A few minutes later, the two police officers deliver the young man to the nearest hospital. The admitting nurse in the ER asks him to sit while she inputs his information. He lunges at her, throws a wild left hook at the air next to her face. The cops grab him, pin his arms behind his back, and slip plastic restraints over his wrists.

The ER resident on call treats the young man for a minor head injury but given his level of intoxication, his attempted assault on a hospital staff member, as well as his impending arrest for driving under the influence, driving to endanger, uprooting a mailbox, and crashing into three vehicles, the medical staff admits him to the hospital. The cops escort him to a room on the third floor, where a nurse hooks him to an IV and a monitor as one of the police officers straps him to his bed. Satisfied that the young man, heavily sedated and his wrists secured, no longer poses a threat to himself or anyone else, the cops leave.

Big mistake.

The young man somehow wriggles out of his restraints, unhooks the IV and monitor, opens the window, and swan dives out. He does a face-plant in a dumpster, breaking his nose, his arm, his ankle, and smashing several ribs. The same two cops, returning to their cruiser in the parking lot, hear the crash coming from the side of the building. Sprinting, they follow the sound, arriving just in time to see the young man, his face a bloody crimson mask, climbing out of the dumpster. He sees the cops, rolls out of the dumpster, hits the ground, and limps away as fast as he can before the first officer grabs him. The young man whirls and punches the cop in the throat. Stunned, the cop falls back. The young man starts running. The second cop catches up to the young man, tackles him, and brings him down onto the blacktop of the parking lot, crunching another of the young man's ribs. The drunk struggles, swears, and spits blood at the cop through his cracked teeth and bleeding lips. The first cop drops onto the young man's back and cuffs his wrists again, this time with metal handcuffs. Then the cops lift the young man and carry him back to the ER, as he squirms, swears, punches, and screams the entire way.

* * *

"He jumped out of a third-floor window?" I ask, incredulous. "Seriously?"

Monique, the lead nurse, stands next to me at the nurses' station in the ER. She's in her forties with a heart-shaped face and eyes that seem to permanently twinkle. Monique's figure is sturdy, her personality large, and her manner direct. She pulls no punches, and she suffers no fools. You do not mess with Monique.

"Uh-huh," Monique says. "After he got away from the police, assaulted the ER intake nurse, and attacked the two police officers."

"He had to be drunk."

She cocks her head with a classic Monique been-there, done-that smirk. "You think?"

I shrug, acknowledging how oblivious and obvious my statement was. "What else is going on with him?"

Monique nods at her clipboard, flips to the next page. "You want the short list or the long list?"

I look over her shoulder and read aloud. "Broken arm, broken ankle, three broken ribs, and a broken nose. Any internal injuries?"

"Nope." Monique offers me the clipboard as if she's the hostess at a five-star restaurant handing me a leather-bound menu. I take it from her and bow slightly.

"I almost forgot," Monique says. "He's a real prick."

"My lucky night," I say.

"Have fun, Doctor Black Cloud...I mean *Tony*."

* * *

I part the curtain separating the ER from an area in the corner. A young man around my age sits upright in a bed. His left wrist is chained to the first rung of the metal frame. He glares at me as I close the curtain. At least I think he glares. Hard to tell since his face is covered in blood.

"Hey," I say, trying to sound as normal as possible, but not quite succeeding. I take another look at his chart, scan his injuries, and decide I'll start with his face. I approach the side of the bed and lean down.

He spits a big viscous bloody loogie. *Splat!* The gob hits my cheek. I step back, wipe away the spittle, and stare at him.

"I took an oath, but I don't have to treat you," I say. "I can send in somebody else. Can't say who that'll be. But it might be someone with less experience and a lot less patience."

The guy tries to bring his arm across his chest toward me but his hand, restrained by the chain, jerks spastically as if it belongs to a puppet. He drops his hand to his side and grunts in frustration and pain.

"So, let's start over," I say. "I'm Doctor Youn."

"Wait," he says. "Did you say Doctor Youn?"

"Yes."

"Are you...*Tony*?"

"What? Uh, yeah. Do I know you?"

"Richie Bayless. We went to high school together."

"Holy crap," I say. "Richie. Man."

"Wow," Richie says, a hint of a smile struggling to make its way through the blood on his face. "What the hell happened to you?"

I laugh. I can't help myself. "I know, right?"

Richie snorts, a kind of bitter laugh. After another small pause, he says, "I'm pretty messed up, huh?"

"I've seen worse," I say.

"How bad am I?" Richie says.

"Put it this way, you're gonna live."

Richie turns his head and mutters, "I was afraid you were gonna say that."

I can't figure out what to say to that, so I pretend I don't hear him. I open a drawer in the supply cart, find a pair of gloves, and begin cleaning the cuts on his face. "I think the last time we saw each other was graduation, right?" I say. "That day seems like an eternity ago. Have our lives really deviated this much in the past nine years?"

"Yeah." Richie winces as I dab at a wound with a medicated cotton swab. His breath reeks of beer and cigarettes. I start swabbing another cut. Richie grimaces. "Ow."

"Sorry," I say.

Richie closes his eyes as I continue to clean him up. "We had some good times back at Greenville High, didn't we? A lot of fun..."

"Parties," I say. "Cruising. Lots of driving around in your VW Rabbit."

"*Lots* of driving around," Richie says, and we both laugh.

Richie studies me for a minute. Then he says, "You changed, Tone. You grew up. Me? It's like I never left high school."

"So, what happened here?"

"Remember Alice Pretzel?"

"Sure. Weren't you two a couple?"

"On again, off again, then a couple years after graduation, we hooked up and she got knocked up. So, we made it official, got married, had another kid, her dad gave me a job working at his auto parts store, life was good. We were like the perfect couple. And then..."

He pauses. I feel the emotion coursing through him.

"I caught her cheating on me," Richie says. "Some guy at her job. Foreman. Big man. She said she was gonna leave me and take the kids. I was not gonna let her take my kids away. I got pissed. I lost it."

"That was tonight," I say.

Richie nods. "I drank a six-pack. For courage. Waiting for her to come home, I kept picturing her with him. Him acting like Dad to my kids. I drank some more. Then she walked in the door and I went off. Threw shit. Broke shit. Screamed at her. Called her a bitch, this, that, I don't know, like I was in some kind of weird black hole. And then..."

He swallows hard, lowers his voice.

"She slapped me. I...I reacted. I slapped her back. I didn't mean to. It was just like reflexes, ya know? She called the cops. One phone call and, pfft, my life ends. I admit it. I...snapped. I...just..."

I stop dabbing at Richie's wounds because he's crying.

"I ran," he says. "I messed everything up. I can't believe it. I'm not gonna see my kids again. I ruined everything."

I look at Richie Bayless, my former high school classmate, sobbing, his head lowered clumsily into his hands, his wrists chained to the frame of his hospital bed. The wind is knocked right out of me. I want to say something to comfort him, but I'm at a loss. I'm not even sure where to look. Richie raises his head and through eyes soaked with tears, with blood crusted on his face, he says, "What could I have done, Tony?"

"I don't know, Richie," I say. "The heat of the moment..."

"I was blind with rage. I wanted to strike back at her..."

For a long time neither of us speaks. Richie drops his head back into his hands and rocks back and forth, sobbing softly. I reach over and rest my hand on his shoulder. "You need to have some X-rays taken, Rich."

Richie opens his eyes and, as if realizing where he is for the first time, looks at his surroundings in this curtained-off area of the emergency room. He looks straight ahead and says, simply, "The decisions you make."

I want to say something wise and helpful. Instead I say nothing.

"If I'd walked away," Richie says. "If I'd been strong enough to make that one right decision, to leave instead of getting drunk and going after her, everything would be different."

The decisions you make.

Those words reverberate as if Richie has screamed them.

"It's not too late to make good decisions," I say, even though it sounds totally lame. "To turn it around."

"For me?" Richie says. "It's pretty late, Tone."

But in the next days at least, during his nearly one-week hospital stay, Richie does make better decisions. He cooperates with every doctor who sees him. He acts courteously to every nurse. He apologizes to the intake nurse he took a swing at.

Richie undergoes orthopedic surgery to repair his broken bones. I sit with him every day and we chat and reminisce. One day I check on Richie after rounding on my patients. He's gone. The nurse on his floor tells me the attending doctor discharged Richie from the hospital into the custody of two uniformed police officers who took him to jail.

I never see Richie again, but I think about our conversations.

He was right. I have changed.

I changed because I wanted to change.

And now I want to become a responsible adult.

I want to be responsible to my peers, my patients, my parents, myself, and my wife.

Yes, my wife.

I want to marry Amy.

The decisions you make.

* * *

Now that I've decided to propose, I join the ranks of the millions of clueless dudes throughout history who've tried to come up with a sufficiently romantic, unclichéd, and hopefully successful way to pop what will certainly be one of the biggest questions of my life. The feared, dreaded, unchartered will-you-marry-me question.

I'm only going to do this once.

I'm determined to do it right.

* * *

I spend a frantic week in the middle of a frigid December telling my parents that I'm going to ask Amy to marry me.

Mom: "Tony, that is wonderful. I'm so proud of you."

Dad: "Thank God. How long you go out? Four years? Finally. Slowpoke. Mommy and I wonder if you gay. Such good news. And Amy is perfect for you. I love her so much. She's not Asian so you will have a hard life, miserable sometimes, but that's OK. You love each other and I love her and she's *perfect*."

I sneak out to dinner with Amy's parents and secretly ask for their daughter's hand. They both cry. On Saturday, I tell Amy that I feel like going for a drive.

"Today? The wind chill is like minus ninety. Let's stay home and watch a movie."

"Oh, OK, great idea, but you know what? I really feel like driving. I'm antsy. I need to get out. I want to show you something. Something I've been meaning to show you, give you, tell you, uh, yeah, let's go." I realized by the time I've gotten to the end of that sentence, I sound unhinged.

Amy confirms this with a puzzled face as she asks, "Are you all right?"

"Me? No, no, yeah, I'm *fine*."

"You are acting so weird. You've been spending a lot of time in the ER. Have you been self-medicating? Doing a little 'one for you, one for me' prescribing?"

"*Hahahahaa!*" I laugh like a self-medicator.

I manage to whisk her away to Saugatuck without further conversation or suspicion on her part. At least I don't think she suspects anything. Once we arrive in the little artsy town we take a walk on the boardwalk along the river, both of us freezing, bundled up to our eyes. I know she's shivering and uncomfortable but she doesn't complain. Finally, I blurt something about her being my soulmate and wanting to spend the rest of my life with her and that she's so great and beautiful.

"Wait, what?" she says. "The wind's kicking up. I couldn't hear you. Plus, I think I lost a couple of toes back there. I feel them bouncing around inside my sock...."

I drop to my knees on the frozen tundra. I look up into a flurry of snow, and in a voice that quivers from equal parts freezing cold and nervous terror, I ask:

"Will you marry me?"

She screams. She says yes. We hug. We kiss. Then, numb from cold and love, we get the hell back inside the warm car. We drive to our favorite restaurant, The Evergreen Grill, an hour and a half away.

To her shocked delight, I've arranged to have our parents and my brother and sister waiting for us. That's when she cries. But that's the good kind of tears. The best kind of tears.

Her dad pops open a bottle of champagne and we all toast. I look at her and my heart fills up. I try not to cry, but I do, only a little. OK, maybe a little more than a little, because I love Amy so much.

I know that I won't always make the right decisions.

But today I did.

6

Finding My Voice

After a weekend conference for general surgery residents—anyone beyond first year—we sit, the original five of us, around a table in the lunchroom dissecting the highs and lows of the conference. Gunner Shelley found the sessions superficial. "Nothing I didn't know or hadn't experienced," she says, nose up, hair flipped back, a true gunner's sexy pose of nonchalant superiority.

"I felt just the opposite," Jessica says. "I found the sessions overwhelming. So much information coming at you. I felt bombarded. Then I got anxious and when I get anxious, I eat. I think I OD'd on Skittles."

"I wanted more war stories," Conrad says, his voice dark and breathy. "I wanted to hear about surgeries gone bad, flesh-eating bacteria, or a schizophrenic coming to the ER with his severed junk in a bag and it has to be reattached. I find that sort of stuff instructive."

"We know," Jessica says. "You're a ghoul."

Superstar Garth, sitting at the head of the table, nursing an iced tea, looks off, distracted, absently playing with his straw.

"Yo, Garth," Conrad says. "What were you and Bledsoe and those other two docs talking about? Looked like you were having an intense conversation."

"Huh?"

"What were you and those guys discussing?"

Garth faces toward us and eyes me directly.

"Nothing," he says, and then looks at Conrad. "Nothing at all, Conrad."

I catch Garth's look at Conrad. But Conrad, too thick to receive Garth's clear-as-day message to change the subject or shut up, presses on.

"Come on," Conrad says. "You guys were talking for like ten minutes. Laughing, slapping each other on the back. Tell us right now or I will hurt you."

All our eyes land on Garth as if he's a reluctant kid and we're brutal stage mothers shoving him forward for his unwanted solo in the spotlight.

Garth waits for a beat, then shrugs, as if to say, *OK, fine, I'll tell them. What the hell*. He spreads his palms on the table.

"We were talking about the future," he says. "And they were saying...heck, I'm not sure how to say this because it's embarrassing, but, fine, you asked. They said to me, 'Well, you know, Garth—we think you've really got it going on. We think you're going to be huge. A high-powered, well-known, big-time plastic surgeon. One of the best in the country. You're gonna change thousands of people's lives, become famous, and retire with a golden scalpel. Yadda, yadda, yadda.' That's what they said."

All the air is sucked out of the room. Especially when I feel everyone looking at me. "What about me? Did they happen to mention the other plastic surgery resident sitting next to you, the doofus who's always number two to your number one?"

That's what I want to say. Luckily, the sensors block that comment before it can spurt out of my mouth and expose what an insecure, bitter, wannabe plastic surgeon I feel like at that particular moment.

Garth, I guess picking up my cue, feels compelled to deal with the proverbial elephant in the room, and goes right for it.

"But, hey, Tony, they're also very well aware of you."

He scrunches his forehead, realizing that didn't come out the way he, or I, might've hoped. Garth tries again, "What I mean is..." He clears his throat, realizing that he's dug himself into a deep pit. "They think you're *terrific*." Then too fast: "They think you're a really good guy and that you have a definite shot of doing well too. They see you becoming, at the very minimum, a reasonably decent plastic surgeon. At *minimum*."

Wow.

A long, painful—achingly painful—silence.

A silence that bruises an internal organ.

"Well," I say at last. "At least they mentioned me."

Our table's obviously too loud laughter rocks the room.

Garth's face burns red. "I'm older," he attempts to explain, trying to salvage the moment. "I have kids. They relate to me. They see me as more mature."

"You're kind of making it worse," Jessica says just above a murmur.

"No, I understand," I say a little too quickly. "It's fine. It's cool. I get it."

I'm bullshitting.

It's actually not fine or cool.

And I don't get it.

* * *

"People think once you have 'Doctor' in front of your name you have it made."

"Ha!" my father says.

The two of us sit in my parents' living room after a Sunday dinner. Amy and my mother have holed themselves up in the kitchen. They insist on doing the dishes themselves so they can hash, rehash, and re-rehash wedding plans. My father expects this and I don't object.

"Easier to become a doctor than *be* a doctor," my father says, picking his teeth with a wooden toothpick. He smiles and adds softly, "Daddy so proud of you. So proud. You're gonna be very skillful surgeon."

"I'm not so sure," I say.

"Oh," my father says and waves those words away like a bad smell. "No doubt."

I scoot to the edge of the couch and lean forward, talking quietly to make sure my mother and Amy can't possibly hear. "What if my training isn't good? Or what if I get sued and lose everything?"

"That the most important thing. Your training. Train well. Work hard. Work very hard. Harder than anyone. You must do that. And you have to take very good care of your patients. You do that and you will not get sued."

I nod, assuming that he's right. But nagging at me like a gnat is the fact that some things are just not in anyone's control. Certainly not mine. My father lays the chewed-up toothpick on the table. I look at that soggy masticated thing, and I can't help but think it's a metaphor for my medical career.

"You know, Daddy's been working thirty years. Daddy's birthed four thousand babies. The whole town. Four *thousand* babies. And never got sued. Why? Daddy takes care of his patients. Always. That's what you will do."

Now he leans in to me, so close our knees bump.

"I have colleague, guy I know, very good doctor. He make one mistake. Whole career. He misdiagnose one patient. One mistake. Boom." He ticks off the results on his fingers. "He get sued, big lawsuit, he lose case in court, he lose license, and"—he makes a face indicating the worst is about to come—"he move whole family to Peoria." He pauses for effect and then says with horror: "*Peoria!*"

We lean back into the couch simultaneously. We sit in silence for several moments.

"Four thousand babies," my father says, and then adds with a sigh, "Just work harder and be careful."

"And," I say, "take care of my patients."

* * *

The thing is, as a second-year resident, I don't really have any patients of my own. The patients belong to the chief residents or the attendings. While I certainly feel responsible when I treat them, I could never claim them as my own patients. I wonder: Does this make me less than a full-fledged doctor? I don't see a way around the system, or that feeling, until I have my own practice. Then one night something happens on the burn unit.

* * *

Often, I work alone with the nurses on the burn unit. I give the more serious "burn codes" to Dr. Winslow, a thirty-year veteran of burn and trauma surgery. He's a tall, haughty, white-haired workout fanatic who blows into the burn unit with a God-like swagger and a mile of attitude. I don't think he likes me. Worse, sometimes I think he doesn't know I even exist.

But until Dr. Winslow struts in like a puffy peacock in a shiny white doctor's coat, I'm in charge. I tend to the most precarious and compromised patients, victims of electrical accidents, industrial explosions, house fires, and even the occasional chemical spill. Screaming ambulances sent from 911 calls take too long for these cases. Most arrive in helicopters.

I hover over each burn victim with exquisite care, attending meticulously, figuring out what fluids and medications to dispense and if a patient should be put on a ventilator. Finally, for better and for worse, I am completely responsible. I start to feel more like a doctor and less like a chief resident's sidekick. I am, for once, more Batman than Robin.

One night near downtown, an explosion rips through a plastics plant, causing a fireball to blow through the main factory floor. Martin, a man working the late shift, is engulfed in flames and suffers burns on over 90 percent of his body. A helicopter brings him to the burn unit. I literally sprint to take care of him, nurses galloping behind. I carefully cut away blackened, still-smoking shreds of clothing. Every inch of his body, except for his face and genitals, has been singed to a sickening brown-yellow pulp. As I assess his burns, Martin blinks. Even that minute movement laces his face with pain.

He manages to whimper, "I know it's bad." He closes his eyes, his breathing coming slowly, haltingly.

My heart races and a sickening feeling settles into the pit of my stomach. I am talking with a man who is likely going to die. People with full thickness burns over 90 percent of their body almost never survive. But there's no time for me to despair. He needs my help *now*.

"Hang in there," I say, touching his cheek gently, one of the few unburned areas on his entire body. He nods, grimaces. I step back and call for a heavy dose of pain medication. A nurse runs a line of morphine into the IV in his arm. We determine that Martin's lungs have been burned on the inside. They will soon start accumulating fluid and he will not be able to breathe. I make a decision then that we have to put Martin on a ventilator. He will be comfortable, but he will not be able to speak, and he will be facing certain death. I calculate, conservatively, that Martin will not last more than a few hours.

My mind races. Sweat trickles down my forehead and into my eyes.

Come on, Tony, is there anything else you can do to help this poor guy live? Think, damn it!

Suddenly, a commotion. A whoosh of a parting curtain. A gust of musk. Dr. Winslow, his white coiffed haircut fluttering, his buff shadow falling ominously over both me and Martin, stands sphinxlike at the corner of the bed. With unnecessary flair, he snaps on his mask and gloves and nods gravely, like he's on stage performing in front of an adoring audience. Dr. Winslow pushes past me like I'm not even there, and assesses everything I've done, checking Martin's medication and grunting low and ominous at his severe condition.

"Well," he says. "You've done all you can, Tony. Where's the family?"

"In the waiting room," a nurse says. "His wife and daughter. She's about ten."

"All right," Dr. Winslow says. "Let's put him on the ventilator now."

Time stops.

In the frame of a half second, I lose my sense of self and space. I alter the definition of myself. I'm no longer a doctor. I've relinquished that somehow. I revert to being a lowly resident, a student relegated to the sidelines, or worse, to the shadows. I'm merely here, displaced, an onlooker. I go back to being Robin to his Batman.

But then the faces of the nurses horseshoed around me blur and someone readies the ventilator. I seem to regain my balance, and then my focus. I look at Martin's sad ruined face and at Dr. Winslow standing over him, his towering presence overwhelming every molecule of this closed-in, trapped little corner of the hospital. I know in my heart that Dr. Winslow's decree to hook Martin to a ventilator immediately, at this moment, is medically right, but morally wrong.

I clear my throat.

"I'm, uh, wondering..." I start haltingly, without conviction, like a recently neutered eunuch. And then, miraculously, I rediscover my confidence. My volume rises and a timbre of authority fills up my voice, almost sounding like the echo of a stronger, wiser, more powerful man. I turn to Dr. Winslow as if everyone else has left the room. "If we put him on the ventilator right now, in all likelihood, he's never going to wake up. I think we should bring in his family first so they can say good-bye."

Winslow frowns. He cups his craggy chin between his thumb and index finger. He looks down, past Martin, it seems, as if studying the pattern in the floor. He raises his head after ten long seconds.

"No," he says. "I don't think so. People want hope. If we bring the family in while he's awake to say good-bye, they're gonna lose all hope that he'll survive."

To my own shock and awe, I don't let it go. I press it. "But this may be their one and only opportunity to say good-bye. Maybe he'll wake up, maybe, but it's very doubtful. We both know he's probably never going to survive this. And then they wouldn't have said good-bye. I think we should give them that chance...."

"No." Dr. Winslow pushes past me, dismissing me with maximum condescension. "No. We need to preserve whatever hope we can."

"But..."

"I said *no*, Doctor Youn!" His final word. He gives a signal to the respiratory therapist next to the ventilator. She catches my eye, holds for a moment, and then gets the machine ready.

I step back, into the shadows, it feels.

Later, a nurse brings Martin's wife and daughter into the room. The instant they see Martin looking like a burned, charred hunk of flesh attached to the ventilator, his breathing labored, unable to react to them, they fall apart, their sobs coming at us in uncontrollable bleats. By then, Dr. Winslow and his ego have packed it in and gone home. After a while, the nurses guide Martin's wife and daughter out of the hospital room and back to the waiting area, where they cling to each other, hanging on to whatever thread of hope they have concocted.

My shift ends and I leave for the night. In my apartment, I don't have the strength to take off my clothes. I collapse onto my bed like a marionette with the strings cut. But I can't sleep. I'm too wired, too on edge, too emotionally exhausted. After a few fitful hours of playing and replaying the scene with Dr. Winslow, the horribly injured Martin, and his poor suffering wife and child, I shower and return to the hospital an hour before my shift. I go to the burn unit.

Martin's bed is empty. I find the nurse on call and she confirms what I fear. Martin died two hours after I left.

I nod, thank her for the information, turn a corner, slam my hand against the wall next to the elevator. I curse. I lean my palms into the wall. I feel my shoulders sag.

His wife. His daughter.

His family never got to say good-bye.

His wife never got to tell her husband that she loved him one last time.

His daughter never got to say one final *I love you* to her daddy.

Nothing I could've done, I tell myself. I couldn't have questioned Dr. Winslow. He's my teacher, my superior. And, oh, yes, by the way, I'm Korean and we don't challenge authority. Not how I was raised.

Except Dr. Winslow was wrong.

I know that in every fiber of my being.

And yes, I can work harder—that's part of my culture too—but that won't help what I need to change in myself.

From now on, I will act like the real physician I have become. These patients will be *my* patients. I have earned the word *Doctor* in front of my name. I will now own it. I respect Dr. Winslow and every resident in this hospital. They are my superiors and my teachers and I defer to their experience and their expertise and I will continue to learn from them every minute of every day. But not one of them is God. They're only playing it.

I say a silent prayer, asking God to give me the strength to be the doctor my patients need me to be.

From now on, I will fight for my opinion, always, especially when I know I'm right.

Otherwise, I am lost.

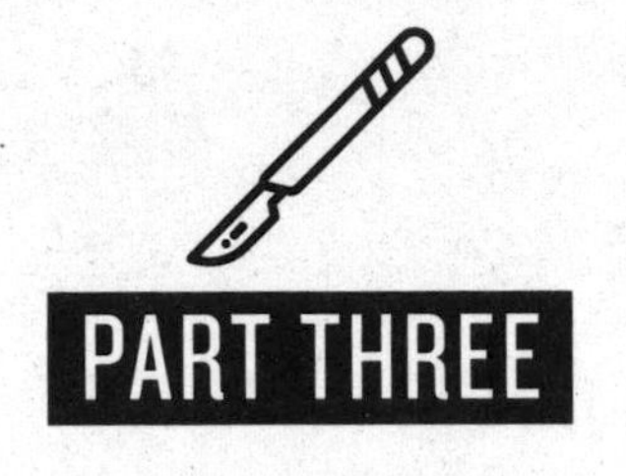

PART THREE

RESIDENCY—YEAR THREE

7

Going Toe to Toe with Death

Year three.

My last year of general surgery before I concentrate on plastic surgery for my final two years of residency.

But those are kind of like dog years, so you have to multiply by seven.

I start to perform more operations on my own—hernia repairs, gallbladder removals, mastectomies. By day I run the surgical ICU under the stern, watchful stare of the surgical intensivist attending, Dr. Phyllis Zorich. She's a large, sullen block of a woman with a tar-black buzz cut, ironically cute dimples dug into her granite cheeks, and no visible trace of a personality. Dr. Zorich, who towers over me, clicks her tongue loudly whenever she's annoyed or impatient. When she's around me, the clicking never stops.

In the ICU we see critical care patients who suffer some type of surgical emergency after an accident—usually a car crash—or a severe illness, such as pancreatitis. Typically, I lead a group of a half dozen or so interns, rounding on the patients, with Dr. Zorich clicking constantly at my side as I talk through each patient's condition, medical concerns, and likely procedures. Once, when I trip up after answering an intern's question, Dr. Zorich jumps in eagerly, bodychecking me into the wall before correcting me. I thank her and apologize.

"I wouldn't have expected you to be up to speed on that information," Dr. Zorich mutters after an endless bout of clicking. "You're not a real surgery resident. You're going into *plastics.*" She exaggerates the word, hanging on the soft *a* and then sniffs as if I've chosen a specialization equivalent to male hustling or selling used cars.

At night, I'm the lead physician covering the ICU. I'm usually accompanied by an intern who follows me like a puppy, while Dr. Zorich thankfully takes her clicking on the road, retiring for the night to what I imagine is her coven, where she lives with her ever-clicking significant other and their clicking children.

In the mornings, looking to let off steam, I seek out Gunner Shelley or Jessica in the cafeteria. I usually don't find either, but invariably bump into Superstar Garth. We compare notes, figuratively and literally, as we prepare for our upcoming five-hour annual "shelf exams," our mandatory multiple-choice in-service exams. Given our insane schedules, nobody expects us to ace these tests, but priding myself on my rep as an academic uber athlete, I still want to bring home the gold for Team Michigan State Grand Rapids on the multiple-choice exam. Last year, putting in about a third of the hours I wanted to, I scored a more than respectable eighty-three. I vow to top that.

"I tried to study last night," Garth says, pouring some coffee. "I couldn't. I just crashed. I'm worried that I might bomb this thing."

He's so lying. This is Garth's passive-aggressive trash talking. He's never failed a thing in his life. I know he put in three hours. Two hours minimum. I managed to squeeze in an hour myself while I was on call.

"Did you study?"

"No, man," I say, yawning for effect, excising the top of a blueberry muffin. "It was a zoo last night. I didn't have a minute." I'll show him I can lie with the best of them.

"Well, the shelfies don't matter anyway," Garth fibs into his coffee cup.

"A total formality," I lie through a mouthful of muffin.

"Garth!"

Click.

"Doctor Ellington, I presume."

The menacing master of condescension has returned.

Dr. Zorich strolls toward us, engulfing the cafeteria in darkness. She pulls up at our table, slaps Garth on the back, and grins malevolently at me, revealing a set of fangs sharp enough to tear through the flesh of an elk.

"Good morning, Doctor Z." Garth returns her grin and rolls his neck, grunting ecstatically as Zorich starts kneading his shoulders like a world-class masseuse.

"Doctor Zorich," I say. "Great to see you."

Click.

"Listen, Doctor Youn," she says, her hands and fingers working the kinks out of Garth's neck. "Would you do us a favor?"

Us?

"Would you mind rounding on Garth's patients? Something I need to discuss with Doctor Ellington. In private."

I stare. She clicks.

"We're only talking three patients. Take you a half hour."

"No, no, that's OK." Garth shifts forward so Dr. Zorich is forced to cut her backrub short. "Tony shouldn't have to round on my patients. I'll do it. We can talk later."

"No, no, no," I say, standing. "Happy to do it."

"You sure?" Garth says, oozing false gratitude. "I owe you."

"Nah," I say. I have to stop myself from adding, *Just tank the shelfies.* Not that I feel any competition with Garth. I ease by Dr.

Zorich, a final deafening *click* at my back threatening to shatter an eardrum.

For the record (not that I care, *really*!), when we do take the tests, I kill without even trying, scoring ninety-six.

Garth, without ever studying—according to him—scores ninety-eight.

* * *

A week later I make a totally unexpected friend for life.

It's a Saturday night when the EMTs pull a sixteen-year-old boy out of an SUV mashed and twisted beyond recognition against the guardrail on the interstate. Miraculously, the majority of his body has escaped serious damage, but the boy has suffered a closed head injury. So while his skull has remained intact, his brain has been bruised and damaged. If the brain bleeds or swells, it can increase the pressure inside the skull. Because bone surrounds the brain, there is no place for the brain to expand. Simply put, if the pressure inside his brain ultimately spikes too high, his brain will herniate—rupture—and the boy will die.

I order a CT scan. As expected, the scan shows a massive traumatic brain injury with pressure rising like a deadly brain tornado. I consult with the neurosurgeon on call. We agree on a course of action: the neurosurgeon will drill a small hole into the boy's skull and insert a catheter into the space around his brain to allow fluid to leak out, resulting, hopefully, in a drop in pressure. Right now my whole world has shrunk to one thing. Keeping the boy alive. We watch him, constantly, his head wired into monitors. We follow his pressure levels moment by moment. We desperately try to lower the pressure through a plethora of measures, including several medications shot through an IV attached to his limp, lifeless arm.

His parents sit at his bedside all day, leaving their watch only for bathroom breaks. His father rarely speaks. He leans forward in his chair, his eyes gazing at the floor, his elbows resting on his knees, his hands folded in front of him as if in prayer. His mother scribbles incessantly in a journal, jotting thoughts, feelings, observations, recording, it seems, every instance of their ordeal. She will later turn her journal into a book.

I catch the mom's eye and bathe in her helplessness and her hope. Of course, I want to assure her that everything will be all right. But in fact I can only hope along with her. Toward the end of their first twenty-four-hour vigil, I'm tempted to ask them to take a few hours off, to go home, shower, and grab a few hours of sleep. But I say nothing. I know they won't leave. I wouldn't either.

The evening of the second day, Dr. Zorich is the doctor on call, the attending physician whom I (the junior resident) will answer to that night. She enters the room, eyes the monitors, studies the pressure levels, offers me the slightest, nearly imperceptible nod of what I, ever the cynical optimist, interpret to be satisfaction. Or at least not annoyed disgust. She heads off for the night, without a single click, reminding me to page her should the boy's condition change.

Days ago, over our morning coffee and bagels, Garth and Jessica say they've heard a rumor that Dr. Zorich is celebrating something special this evening. We take guesses: a major birthday (Fifty? Sixty? Seventy? Two hundred?); her wedding anniversary (a stretch); winning Dominatrix of the Year (strong possibility). Sometime after midnight, I ease into the call room. I'm about to cuddle up with my pillow and try to snatch a couple of hours of sleep when my pager whirs. I sprint to the nurses' station and find the nurse who paged me. "His pressures are going up," she says, clearly worried.

"Is the tube still working?" I say, the words tumbling out unchecked.

"The ventricular catheter doesn't seem to be helping." The nurse speaks slowly, with exaggerated patience, as if English is not my first language.

"I want a CT scan," I say. "Let's bring him now. Right away."

I have to determine the condition of his brain, I know that much. I need to make sure he hasn't developed bleeding around his brain, causing his pressures to spike. And I need to follow protocol.

I call Dr. Zorich.

Her phone goes straight to voice mail.

I call again.

Again, straight to voice mail.

I leave an urgent message.

I try her pager.

I check the boy's pressures.

They've skyrocketed.

If I don't do something fast, we're going to lose him. I flash on having to tell his silent dad and his writing mom that I let their boy die.

The nurses unhook him from the monitors and wheel him toward the CT scanner. I look at my watch. Ten minutes since I called Dr. Zorich. I call her again. Voicemail.

I check the scan as he's wheeled back to the surgical ICU. At that instant, I fear that the boy's brain is about to herniate.

Thank God! The CT scan shows no new bleed or lesion.

That's the good news. Bad news is the pressures inside his skull are still through the roof. If I don't do something to relieve the pressure, his brain is going to herniate and he will die.

I try Dr. Zorich. Again.

Voice mail.

I look at my watch.

Nineteen minutes. No return call.

Not uncommon. Sometimes doctors will take up to twenty minutes to return a call, even an urgent one.

I don't have that kind of time. I cannot sit and wait for Dr. Zorich. I have to do something. I have to make a decision right now, on my own, or this poor boy will crash and burn. I look at the nurse who stands poised at my side, her face lined in anticipation.

"Let's hyperventilate him," I say.

She hesitates. "Hyperventilate..."

"Yes. Now. Immediately."

"What's happening?"

The mom.

She gets to her feet for what seems like the first time in three days. Her legs wobble and she sways slightly. The dad stands beside her, supporting her with one hand on her back, holding her other hand with his.

"He's going to be all right," I say, wanting that more than anything, fighting to believe it. "Just, please, be calm, and sit down, or if you'd rather go into the waiting room...."

"No," the dad says, gently assisting his wife back down to her chair. He sits next to her, heavily, his hand still entwined in hers.

Their son's pressures continue to rise. I envision his pupils dilating as his brain herniates out of his skull and then his heart flatlining. Sweat beads on my forehead. A wave of nausea fills my stomach. I taste bile in the back of my throat.

I need to do something. Now.

"Let's start Mannitol. Twenty-five grams. Please start it *now*!"

The nurse hesitates. "Are you sure?"

"Yes, I am! Just do it!"

The nurse switches the bags attached to the boy's IV and begins the Mannitol. We wait, all of us, the trauma team and me, our midnight leader, glancing at the glowing face of my phone praying for Dr. Zorich to ring. I switch the phone to vibrate. I'm so on edge that the sudden jangling of a cell phone would unhinge me so much I might scream.

We watch the result of the Mannitol. We study the pressure level like military personnel tracking drone strike patterns. We watch in silence, no one daring to speak, no one daring to *move*. The only sound is the *beep, beep, beep* of his heart rate, as minutes drag on.

And then the pressure level drops.

Slightly.

And then it drops again—slightly.

"It's working," someone says. A nurse? An intern? I don't look.

"Not enough," I say. I keep my eyes riveted on the pressure level. I poke my cell phone out of my pocket and start to dial Dr. Zorich. I stop. I tell myself, *She's not calling, Tony. This is on you, Tony. You got this.*

Something shifts in my brain like a piece of a jigsaw puzzle fitting perfectly into the big picture. A recent memory, a familiar calculation, a clear visualization. Suddenly, I know.

"Give him another dose," I say. "Double it."

"Double?"

"*Yes*. Now."

I'm pushing the limit, I warn myself.

I have to, I answer back.

I shut everything out. The images in front of me shimmy and blur. The sounds around me dissolve into a low, distant buzz. And then, gradually, the world comes back into focus. Bodies in motion, feet slapping on the floor, the swish and snap of plastic curtains opening, closing, the wiggle of the IV tubing as the nurse detaches the bag with the previous dose and attaches the new double dose. We wait. My heart thumps in time to the hum of the monitor wired to the young boy's brain. We wait. And then we see...

The pressures dropping.

Big time.

Our collective breath exhaling overpowers the room. I feel as if the floor is tilting. I suddenly realize, as if I've been slapped, that the boy has escaped danger. He has escaped with his life. We went toe-to-toe with death, and kicked him to the curb.

Drifting back into his hospital room, the dad leaps from his chair and pumps my hand. The mom, tears flowing down her cheeks, engulfs me in her trembling arms.

Afterward, I teeter exhausted and disoriented toward the call room with this thought raging, pounding through my head: *He almost herniated. We almost lost him.*

Suddenly, I realize that my phone is vibrating in my pocket.

Dr. Zorich. Calling for the third time.

I never heard or felt the other two calls.

I answer. "Doctor Zorich, it's Tony. Sorry, I just..."

"I heard," she says, and pauses and holds.

I wait for the click disapproval.

It never comes.

Finally, she speaks:

"Get some sleep."

* * *

The following morning, I sit at breakfast with Garth. We share a table in the corner away from sunlight, like vampires in white coats who've just emerged from their coffins. My eyes burn from getting exactly no sleep. I pick at my bagel, abandon it. I consider my coffee, sip it, but it's like trying to chug down mud mixed with motor oil. I push it away. I pick at my bagel again.

"I don't think I would've been able to do what you did," Garth says, scraping his toast with the edge of his plastic knife, the sound ripping into my head like a claw. "I would've frozen."

"You would've done the same thing," I say.

"Honestly? I don't know."

"You would. Instinct takes over. Reflex."

"But how about the dose? That's not reflex. That's knowledge. How did you know to double it?"

I look at him, puzzled and confused. *That* he should know.

"The shelfies," I say. "It was on the exam."

His mouth funnels into a circle. "I don't remember that."

"Must've been the one question you got wrong."

He starts to laugh, then looks off and slams his mouth shut, swallowing his voice. I turn and see Dr. Zorich framed in the doorway of the cafeteria. She sees us, wiggles a tiny wave, and strides toward us. I ball up my napkin and toss it into the middle of my tray, ready for a barrage of clicking and contempt.

"I'll leave you two alone," I say, starting to stand.

"Tony," Dr. Zorich says. The timbre of her voice descends like two weights lowered onto my shoulders, flattening them, and paralyzing me.

"I know we spoke on the phone, but I wanted to talk to you in person."

I catch Garth's worried look, then blink into Dr. Zorich's blinding stare. Incredibly, she has turned her back on Garth. And then, her lips contort into not exactly a smile, but into a shape that seems sort of warm and welcoming. For a moment I think I'm hallucinating, finally descending into sleep-deprived madness.

"Last night," she says, and wags her head, searching for the right word, phrase, and inflexion.

"Impressive," she finally says, with a nod. "Great job."

"Thank you," I manage to spurt out.

"Especially for you, a plastic surgery resident. Very unexpected."

She frowns at Garth, realizing she has nothing to say to him and probably has said too much to me. Then, in what I consider the ultimate act of camaraderie and possibly acceptance, she tears off a piece of my picked-at bagel and pops it into her mouth.

"Carry on," she says, charging toward the door like a fullback plowing into the end zone.

8

Sue Me

I begin meeting my dad once a week in Grand Rapids for dinner, a couple of doctors talking shop. My dad sits across from me, his back ramrod straight, his chest puffed out, reveling in war stories from his practice, expounding on his greatest triumphs, his legacy of birthing a whole generation of children, his deepest satisfaction delivering a couple's children, and then their children's children.

"I birth thousands of babies, thousands," he dives into his weekly trope, his energy high, his voice loud and lively, drawing attention to our table. "Daddy birth whole *town*."

A month or two into our regular dinner routine, Dad hints at retirement. "Daddy getting older. Babies always get born *in the middle of the night*. Why? What is that? My babies can't wait for morning? I'm getting too old, Tony. Hard on my body. Very hard. Can't cheat time."

Gradually, my dad takes his first official step toward hanging up his ob-gyn stirrups for good. He stops delivering babies.

"I feel old, but I still young," he says, perusing the menu at his favorite restaurant, Red Lobster, before settling on his usual, the plate of lake perch. He lays his menu down with a sharp whack of plastic. "I have money in bank. Nest egg. Good financial plan. Mommy and Daddy talk. We think retire while Daddy's *young*. Stay ahead of the game. Couple years more, I'm out. Then go on a cruise, golf with friends." An exaggerated wink. "Play with many adorable grandchildren. *Live*."

He slowly begins dropping the *R* word to his longtime patients, preparing them for his departure and promising a smooth transition to his successor, whoever that will be, when the time comes. Which is, he assures them, at least two years away.

And then one month he cancels dinner, offering no explanation. A conflict, my mom tells me. She doesn't sound really convincing.

The following month he cancels again, this time muttering vaguely through the phone that he's not feeling well.

The next month, he and my mom meet me for dinner together, a surprise since I wasn't expecting her to join us. The three of us sit quietly at Red Lobster. We hardly speak. My father is a little slumped, he looks tired as he absently pats his menu, pretending to study the list of entrées, a look of fake concentration on his face, since he has this menu memorized. Not to mention he orders the same thing every time.

Finally, he lays down his menu carefully, folds his hands, and stares off, a blank look shading his eyes. He seems smaller somehow, distracted.

"The usual?" I ask him. "You having the lake perch?"

"No," he says, softly, distantly. "Too much food. Enough for two people. Just a cup of clam chowder for me."

"Really? You sure? I'm paying."

"So cold in here," he says, his voice cracking. "I tell them to turn down the air. Like icebox. Who can eat?"

My dad pushes himself away from the table, his chair falling over with a clatter. He grunts, picks it up, and trudges toward the hostess standing at the podium. He gestures wildly and then camps under a vent, fluttering his index finger in a windshield wiper motion as if conducting an invisible orchestra in the ceiling.

"What's the matter with him?" I ask my mom. "He's acting weird."

"He's not feeling himself." My mother clears her throat. "Because, well, you know..."

She skids to a stop midsentence.

"What?" I say.

"Daddy's being sued."

"*What?*"

His dark destiny.

The lifelong source of his pride.

Crushed. Destroyed.

"He can't sleep," my mother says. "Grumpy all the time, so stressed, always in bad mood."

"What happened?"

The suit came out of nowhere, my mom explains, a sneak attack, an ambush.

The patient's lawyers have hit him with a case that occurred years ago, just slipping under the statute of limitations.

A couple whose child had fallen into the autism spectrum claims that my father's delivery of their baby caused the disease. The couple is suing for malpractice.

"That's frivolous," I say to my mom. "It's beyond that. It's ridiculous. This case will be thrown out of court in a heartbeat."

"Anyone can sue anybody," my mother says so quietly I have to lean across the table to hear.

"He has malpractice insurance, right?"

"Yes. But he's never been sued. So he never thought to get much protection. His insurance only covers one hundred thousand dollars."

I'm afraid to ask the next question. But I have to. I look away, then back at my mother. "How much are they suing him for?"

My mother hesitates, clearly uncomfortable, demurely patting her chin with her napkin. "A lot more than one hundred thousand dollars."

"How much?"

"Millions," she says barely above a whisper.

* * *

My father suspends our monthly dinners. I call the house often but my mother says he's out or taking a nap. We rarely speak. My mother becomes his mouthpiece, his protector, his firewall. The few times I do see him he seems reflective, sad, disoriented, and strangely diminutive. It's like he's aged a decade in six weeks. I don't know this man. My dad was almost a mythical figure to me, a larger-than-life superhero, the stoical face of an immigrant from the poorest part of Korea who arrived with literally nothing, but thrived. To me, my dad personified power, resolve, and fiery energy. This man—the man who slouches around our family home now like an old tired ghost of himself—has become diminished, a shell of the image I've held in my mind my entire life. He flits from room to room like a wounded bird, never landing in one place. My father has become fragile. Even worse, he seems broken.

One day, sitting in the kitchen with my mother as I sip lemonade and she sorts through a stack of mail, I ask how the lawsuit is going.

"Not good," she says. "Dragging out. Oh. You're gonna be getting some mail addressed to me at your apartment."

"Why?"

She shrugs, avoids my eyes. "Daddy and I are separating."

I feel kicked in the gut. My glass nearly slips through my hands.

"You're *separating*?"

"Yes. We're getting a divorce."

This is too much. I wrap my arms around my stomach. I feel myself weaving. I honestly think I may retch.

My mother looks up from sorting the mail. "Oh, no, no. Not what you think. Don't worry. We love each other and everything is fine."

"Fine? Everything is *fine*?"

"Yes. We're divorcing until this lawsuit gets settled. Better that way. Our attorney says we should move everything into my name. Otherwise..."

She swallows, and peers through the kitchen window.

"Otherwise, we will have nothing. No money. We will be—what's the word?—*destitute.*"

Later that day, my father finally makes a cameo appearance, shuffling into the kitchen from somewhere in the back of the house. I tell him that Mom has explained about their impending divorce.

"Better this way," he says. "Now when I'm old and decrepit, you and your brother and your sister will at least have something so you will be able to take care of me."

"That's a comforting thought," I say, feeling exactly the opposite of comfort.

"Divorcing on paper only," my mother reminds me.

"Yes," my father says. "Not real. But, you know, OK, *real.*"

Their divorce and the upcoming lawsuit shakes me to the core of my soul. Thoughts racing, I find sleep elusive and often impossible. I can't focus, can't concentrate, like the ground is constantly shifting under me, and I'm afraid I'm going to get sucked into the black hole beneath it. I can't imagine how my parents must feel. Family is their foundation. To destroy that, even as a formality, makes me feel as if we've been hit by a bomb.

"Everything's turned upside down," I tell Amy one night. "My father loves being a doctor. It's always been this idyllic career. Hell, it was the only career worth anything. And now that career is destroying him."

"It's more than his career," Amy says. "It's his identity."

"In our culture we talk about saving face or losing face, right?"

"I know."

"Well, my father has lost everything. He's completely humiliated. He's lost face."

"But he will survive the lawsuit," Amy says. "I know he will."

"He will," I say. "But I don't know how he will survive the humiliation."

* * *

The attorney assigned by my father's insurance company urges him to seek an additional opinion, someone who can provide impartial testimony to help him make his case. My father contacts several doctors he knows to stand with him, asking if they will serve as expert witnesses. Every single one turns him down. He's devastated. We all are. Desperate, he cold calls a neonatologist at a well-known distant hospital. In his broken English, this now broken man blurts his plea: "Thank you for taking my call. You don't know me, but I need your help. I am ob-gyn in small town. I am getting sued. I have done nothing wrong. Can you please help me?"

To his shock, the neonatologist, a woman he's never met, says simply, "Let me review your case."

A week later she calls back and says with surprising fury in her voice, "Doctor Youn, I've reviewed your case. You did absolutely nothing wrong. I'm going to speak on your behalf and I'm going to get you out of this."

We breathe a sigh of cautiously optimistic hope.

* * *

Several months and several thousand dollars in legal fees later, the couple drops the case against my father before it ever gets to court. My father, though vindicated, remains shaken, his belief in the sanctity of being a doctor, of working hard, of living a life of care and service to the community, ruined forever. Two years earlier than planned, he announces his retirement. My mom chooses a date for a small party at the hospital. A week or so before the party, my father wants to meet for dinner at Red Lobster.

I arrive a few minutes late and find my parents sitting at their favorite table by the window in the back. My father rises to greet me. He smiles, pats me on the back. He seems happier, his posture is back to normal, and he appears to have some life back in his eyes. He seems almost himself again.

"Sit down, sit down," he says. "How about some champagne?"

"Wow, sure."

"This is the good stuff," he says, pouring me a glass.

"I didn't realize Red Lobster even had champagne," I say.

"No. I bring from home."

"You're in a good mood."

"Very good mood. Lawsuit behind, retirement ahead. Plus..." He raises his glass. "A toast."

My mom and I raise our glasses.

"To my beautiful new wife."

My parents clink glasses and drink. Confused, I suspend my champagne flute in midair, my hand gripping the stem. "I don't understand...."

"We got remarried today," my father says. "We just came from justice of the peace. No more divorce."

"I can't keep up with you two newlyweds," I say.

"I know," my dad says, laughing. "Always something, huh? Exciting to have new bride."

I shake my head and sip the champagne. "Anything else you want to tell me? Any other bombshells?"

"Yes," my mother says.

"Yes?" I say.

"Yes," my father says. "We're moving to California."

"What? When?"

My father shrugs, sips. "Three weeks."

* * *

My parents anticipate that no more than thirty people will attend my father's retirement party at the hospital. Several hundred people show up, packing the room my mom reserved. It feels as if the whole town of Greenville has come out to honor my father, barraging him with nonstop speeches, testimonials, embraces, thanks, gifts, an immeasurable outpouring of love. Former nurses, staff, and patients—entire families—offer my dad their heartfelt gratitude for bringing them and their kids into the world. I hang back with Amy, watching my father accept everyone's warm and loving thoughts. And I can see that he is both moved and overwhelmed.

The day after the party, my parents throw themselves into cleaning out our old house. They pack up everything they will bring to California and sell or give away the rest. On the day the moving van arrives, the house is empty but still not sold. They don't care. They are in a hurry to leave. In my mind, my dad has been completely exonerated. The accusation against him resulted in a paper-thin lawsuit without even the legs to carry it into a courtroom. But to my dad, the lawsuit will forever be a blot on his legacy, an indelible dark stain that he can never erase.

I drive my parents to the airport. We speak little on the way. I want to think of this as a new start for them. And it is; they'll be living in the land of permanent sunshine, endless blue skies, and Disneyland, near relatives in Orange County. But the silence in the car weighs heavy with sadness. I can sense a hint of defeat, a kind of retreat.

At the curb, I unload their luggage. I hug my mom. She clings to me with surprising fervor and I choke up as she starts to cry.

"New beginning," my dad says and then he hugs me too. We break our embrace. I wave to them as they disappear into the terminal. I get into the car and then the wave of sadness hits me. I cry, feeling the loss of my childhood, the loss of the home that I saw as my anchor, and suddenly a loss of innocence. I finally settle myself with a deep breath and drive away from the curb.

I'm about to begin my fourth year of residency, and for the first time since choosing to become a doctor, I have witnessed the dark underbelly of my profession, my passion, my calling. I will come to learn that all doctors live with some fear of being sued. While some live in constant and very real dread. I doubt any doctor will take being sued more personally than my dad, nor will any doctor take the hit so hard. That ridiculous, meritless lawsuit crushed my dad's spirit and broke his heart.

I wonder if it will someday do the same to me.

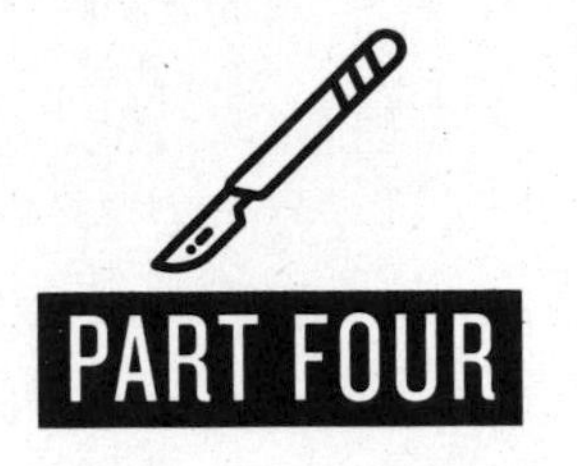

PART FOUR

RESIDENCY—YEAR FOUR

9

Dad Can Dance

I call our wedding the event of the year.

"The event of the *year*? That's *it*?"

Amy.

Sitting across from me at the kitchen table.

Head tilted.

Lips pursed.

Shooting me the stink eye.

"It's not the event of your *life*?"

"No, yeah, it is, I mean, it is *the* most important event of my life, all-time, nothing comes close, well, OK, it's tied, I guess you would have to say, with my funeral, but not really because I won't be there to enjoy that...."

Now she's laughing and shaking her head.

"I'm letting you off the hook because you're so cute when you're flustered. Grab a red pen. We have to winnow down this guest list."

She frowns at the columns of names we've printed out on an Excel spreadsheet. So far we're planning to invite two hundred people to our wedding. So far.

"Do we have to invite all your relatives from Korea?"

"Oh, yeah. Absolutely. But don't worry. They're not gonna come."

They come. Every single one. Apparently, they wouldn't miss the event of the year. I mean, of my *life*.

We marry at the Kirk in the Hills, a massive, imposing stone church in Bloomfield Hills, Michigan, where Amy's parents are members. The first time Amy and I drive onto the church grounds, with the church looming above us majestically like a cathedral somewhere in Europe, its spire cutting through the gray mist, I feel as if I've entered a different world in a previous century.

The wedding is everything we've dreamed, not only a celebration of our marriage but a confluence of our friends and a melding of two cultures. A group of our classmates from medical school are there in all their glory, including the reunion of Tim, James, and Ricky, my closest friends and housemates, the guys who saved my social life and my sanity. Without them, I never would've survived medical school. Superstar Garth and his wife Mrs. Superstar attend, along with the rest of the current gang of five, the walking exhausted, refugees from our three years of residency. My grandparents—my father's parents—come all the way from Korea. My brother is there. My sister, whom I miss dearly since she moved to San Francisco, flies in. Duke, the other remaining member of my band Migration, shows up and by prearrangement brings his trusty guitar. Friends from elementary school and high school come. My first girlfriend comes. It's like taking a stroll down Memory Lane with a who's who of my entire life.

After the emotional ceremony at the epic church, during which I barely hold back tears (and Amy and my mother-in-law don't), we head to the reception hall in downtown Birmingham. My Korean relatives, used to weddings being quiet, sedate affairs ending after a modest dinner, are unprepared for the raucous—and seemingly endless—partying that extends well beyond midnight, all the way into the "hour of the wolf." At first they seem confused, but then they go with the program and throw themselves into the festivities, mobbing the dance floor as only Korean relatives can.

At one point, Duke and I strap on our guitars and with Duke accompanying me, I play and sing "Brown-Eyed Girl" to Amy, then we launch into "Margaritaville" and a wild version of "Southern Cross." During that song, my dad does something I've never seen. So recently ripped apart by that devastating lawsuit, he literally shakes off whatever lasting, ill effects he feels, drags my mom onto the dance floor, and he dances. No, actually, he *dances.* At least I think that's what he's doing. Either that or he is having some sort of seizure. Contorting his face and biting his lower lip like every klutzy white guy in captivity, he bends his arms at ninety-degree angles, slices the air like a robot gone haywire, and shuffles his feet as if trying to stamp out a dozen burning cigarettes. His rhythm is, putting it kindly, eccentric. But it doesn't matter to him, to my mom, or to me. All I care about—all I see–is his smile.

That smile. Flashing and fastened in a wide gleeful gleaming grill of sheer unabashed joy, that smile tells me he's OK. I haven't seen it in awhile, and I realize how much I missed it. And as he holds his smile, he dances, swiveling and spinning awkwardly and violently. I fear he is about to screw himself into the floor, or possibly knock somebody out. But as he rotates and dips and does some crazy knee bend, he catches my eye and gives me a thumbs-up. I feel the pain that he's been holding and hope it's melting away in gleeful herky-jerky spasms.

I look over at Amy, this wonderful woman who, for some reason I still can't fathom, has agreed to be my wife. She is the most beautiful woman I've ever seen and will ever see. Spinning and dancing like a whirling dervish, I realize how good God has been to me, to my entire family. And for the second time in the past two hours, I feel myself tearing up.

10

Fixing Faces

I see faces.

Broken, torn, shattered, disfigured, mashed, mauled, and mutilated from horse kicks, dog bites, fistfights, car wrecks, bottles smashed across them, baseball bats hammered into them, knives slashed through them.

I don't see these faces as ravaged remains. I see them repaired and new. I see them fixed and perfect.

To me these faces are jigsaw puzzles.

I approach each one—even the faces torn wide open with flaps of skin dangling or tissue missing—as a complex problem I must and will solve.

How am I going to turn this tortured mangled mass of blood and skin and fat and cartilage back into a person's *face*?

How can I give this person their life back?

I want the challenge. I take the challenge gladly, even joyfully. I have heard others murmur that I perform miracles. I tell them I'm only putting together puzzles.

As a first-year plastic surgery resident, I fix hundreds of faces, perhaps more than a thousand. I fix them mostly in the emergency room. I fix them on the spot. I have a goal and a mission. I want to repair each face so perfectly that the next day when my boss, the plastic surgery residency director Dr. Bolek, arrives to fix my fixes, he will look at my work, evaluate my repair, and say, simply, "You left nothing for me to do but remove the stitches."

* * *

I learn by doing. I do everything I can. But sometimes I can do nothing. I work in the realm of the hopeful and the hopeless, the sad, the surreal, and even the delusional.

* * *

The hopeless/hopeful...

I care for a woman who has been savaged by flesh-eating bacteria. I work to save first her life and then her skin. Miraculously, the woman survives, but the infection has completely eaten away her groin and inner thighs. I do my best. I rebuild, I restore, I reshape, I reconstruct. Though she will be diminished and somewhat misshapen, with physical therapy, rehabilitation, medication, love, support, and time, the woman, I believe, will be able to resume living her life.

A few months after I discharge her from the hospital, she returns for a follow-up visit at the plastic surgery resident clinic where I work. She's gone from the jaws of death and disastrous disfigurement to looking good, flush, healthy, *alive*. Her wounds are healing. This is one of my happiest moments as a doctor. I am very hopeful. She manages to walk, with difficulty. Beaming, she leans in to me and whispers:

"When can I start having sex?"

* * *

The sad...

I turn down my first patient. A man arrives in the ER in severe distress. I ask him what's going on. He winces and then he drops his pants. I stare, stifling a horrified, creeped-out shout with a cough, a move that's a must in any good doctor's bag of tricks. His genitals are covered by a clump of warts resembling the head of a cauliflower. Many heads of cauliflower. To remove this mass of cauliflower warts, I will have to burn them off. I hesitate. I recall something I read studying for exams about the dangers of smoke rising from burning off genital warts. If I remember correctly, breathing in the fumes can cause genital warts to form *in your throat*.

I visualize trying to tell Amy how I got a cabbage patch growing in my throat. It's a conversation I want to avoid at all costs.

I seek out my boss, Dr. Bolek, who oversees my work in the clinic. I want to make sure I've got this right.

"Can happen," Dr. Bolek says. "Definitely. Extremely nasty. Could be life-threatening too."

"And, I assume, that wearing a surgical mask..."

"Yeah, like that'll help. Tony, the fumes will bypass the mask. A mask is useless."

I absently caress my throat and swallow. I swear I feel some baby cauliflower shoots sprouting already in there. "What do I do?"

"Well, you can turn him down and refer him to another doctor. That's always an option. It's your call."

For some reason, I didn't know this. Or if I knew it, I subconsciously told myself I'd never turn anyone down. Ever. Under any circumstances. But genital warts forming in my *throat*?

Do no harm. One of the first things learned in medical school. Do no harm to *patients.* But does this include do no harm to me, *the caregiver*?

I refer the patient to another doctor.

To this day, I feel a twinge of guilt when I think about him.

* * *

The surreal...

A woman arrives in the ER with a nasty two-inch cut on her cheek. Apparently, during an argument, her boyfriend slashed her with a bottle. We envision creepy strangers in dark alleyways when we think of assault. But the greatest danger is in our homes. From our supposed loved ones.

The woman is nervous, even hyper, possibly on drugs. When I approach her bedside in the ER, two nurses part. I see they have been restraining her. As I examine the condition of the cut, the woman recoils. My heart sinks. I can't even imagine the terrible abuse she's been through. I try to put her at ease.

"Well, there's good news," I tell her. "The cut isn't too deep. I'll be able to fix you up with a few sutures."

The woman glares at me. "Sutures?"

"Yes," I say, giving my best warm, calm, reassuring doctor smile.

"I thought plastic surgeons used *plastic*. Are you some kind of quack? I thought you were a plastic surgeon. I don't want no sutures. I want plastic. I'm leaving!"

She swings her legs off the bed and bolts out of the ER.

I stand glued to my spot too stunned to stop her.

* * *

The delusional...

One guy, Bill, scares the crap out of me. He calls the plastic surgery clinic one day and insists on speaking to me. When I take his call, he flips out, accusing me of having an affair with his wife, whom he insists is one of my patients. He threatens to send his "boys" after me and suggests that it may not be the best idea to start my car. I don't know this Bill guy, I've never heard of his wife—she isn't a patient—and I have no idea why he chose to call me. When I tell him all this, he laughs maniacally, tells me I'm lying, says his boys are on the way and that I'm a dead man.

I've seen *The Godfather* too many times and I'm scared as hell, so I call the police. A police officer shows up at the clinic and attempts to calm me down. The police eventually trace Bill's call to a local nursing home and assure me that while they can't identify Bill specifically, they're pretty sure he's over seventy and suffering from dementia.

A visit from the police doesn't stop Bill from calling me again and again, always claiming I'm having an affair with his wife and promising to send the boys to kill me.

Unfortunately, Bill serves as a precursor of things to come.

PART FIVE

RESIDENCY—YEAR FIVE

11

Island Fever

As my final year of residency begins, Dr. Bolek dangles a prize in front of Garth and me, the two senior plastic surgery residents—a "mission" trip to Thailand. The prizewinner will spend a week working in a clinic performing plastic surgery on little kids, receiving invaluable experience, providing a surefire game changer on a résumé, and possibly punching our ticket all the way to heaven. Unfortunately, Dr. Bolek can take only one of us to Thailand. After much deliberation and soul searching, he decides on Garth. The Chosen One. The Superstar. Big shock. OK, I made up the part about the deliberating and soul searching. I'm sure it took him all of two seconds to make that decision.

Good news, though. While Garth is saving small children in Thailand and earning points toward his future sainthood, I will not be languishing, forgotten, in Grand Rapids. I have won my own trip, a consolation prize of sorts. I too will be hitting the road, all expenses paid, not to a trip on the other side of the world, but to a plastic surgery conference, in Tortola.

"*Where?*" Amy says.

"Tortola. It's an island. Part of the British Virgin Islands. I think. Not positive. Pretty sure it's civilized. Or at least inhabited. We're going to love it."

"We?"

"Yeah. You think I'm going there alone? No way. Remember those vows we made not that long ago?"

"Vaguely."

"Yeah, well, through thick or thin, sickness and in health, all that, or whatever I said in that moment of weakness. Anyway, we're both going."

"Well, in that case, I better get a really cute new bathing suit," she says, hugging me.

Unfortunately, Amy has a scheduling conflict and won't be able to join me in Tortola until the third day of the trip. Arriving with a few other shell-shocked stragglers, we are crammed sardinelike into an ancient, rickety prop job. We touch down at what I can't in good conscience call an airport—airports have massive runways; we land on what looks like a long driveway. I rent a mini beat-up SUV equipped with four-wheel drive, a must, I'm told by the rental agent, a bored islander in a tank top and a swimsuit. I will need a four-wheel drive to negotiate what he calls "bad mountain roads that disappear into nothing." I have a moment of hesitation, imagining myself disappearing into nothing. But then I rally and tell myself that this will be fine, because I have a plan.

Room service, minibar, and on-demand movies. I'm not leaving the hotel room until Amy arrives. That's my plan. And I'm sticking to it.

I wake up too late for breakfast and decide I have to at least make an appearance at the conference. Yes, it's a deviation from the plan. But since I'm being comped for the meeting and the hotel, I do feel obliged. I find a seat at the back of the first session and dutifully scribble notes that I doubt (correctly, I might add) I will ever look at. But at least if anyone asks, I'll have proof that I did venture out of my hotel room. I look around the conference room, not knowing a soul, and feel ridiculously out of place, like a vegan who accidentally wandered into a weeklong carnivore's convention. I have no business here, the only snot-nosed resident among thirty highly regarded, real-life plastic surgeons. Mercifully, the morning session ends. I frantically stow my notes into my briefcase, planning to spend the next two days barricaded in my hotel room. I'm about to exit the conference room when two men close in on me. I'm sure I'm going to be busted, revealed for the no-nothing novice I am, and escorted from the building.

But no.

They introduce themselves. Quite politely.

Not only are they plastic surgeons, but they are leaders in the field, doctors whose work and reputations I know and admire. I work hard to disguise the surprise I feel that they're even talking to me. We strike up a conversation and head over to the buffet lunch together. We arrange to meet afterward at the beach. Lazing on lounge chairs that rest on sand the color and consistency of snow, beneath the bluest sky I've ever seen, sipping frosty cocktails, I mutter, "I could get used to this." The remark elicits grunts of agreement. That night we meet for dinner, then at breakfast in the morning, and then we attend a couple of sessions together, until we're back on the beach the next afternoon, practically BFFs.

"Tonight, we're all going to Bob's," one of my new, much more brilliant, much more successful friends tells me, eyes closed, his suntan lotion-slathered face angled into the sun. "I'll get you directions."

"You have a four-wheel drive, right?" another new friend says.

"Yes."

"You'll need it."

I vacillate wildly between excited and terrified.

* * *

I drive into the sky.

At least that's how it feels.

Hugging the left side of the twisting road, which seems not much wider than a number two pencil, I steer my tiny, wobbly SUV in what feels like a never-ending upward loop, doing my best not to look down. At one point, I inadvertently catch sight of the crisp pale blue ocean a million miles below, as flat and clear as a sheet of ice. I grip the steering wheel until I am literally white-knuckling and puddling with sweat. The SUV putters like a lawn mower. More than once I picture myself losing control and cartwheeling over the side of the cliff, my SUV flipping over and crushing me to a pulp against the jagged rocks or plunging into the blue abyss, drowning me in that vast blue sea that right now doesn't even ripple. Finally, I come to an unmarked road in the middle of a jungle and, following my directions, turn onto it, and begin climbing another steep hill. I feel like I'm ascending Mount Everest without a Sherpa.

Abruptly, out of the mist, a contemporary boxy white house posing on concrete stilts appears before me. Five or six SUVs line the side of the road. I park my exhausted beater behind the last car and, as I walk toward the house, I follow the utterly spectacular panoramic view of the Atlantic jutting below a glass-enclosed wraparound deck. At the front door, I search for a doorbell. Then I realize that the door is open. I edge inside, mumbling a nearly inaudible, "Hello." My two new friends, hands lovingly caressing bottles of Caribbean beer, see me and wave. They seem remarkably happy to see me. I join them in a living room with scuffed hardwood floors and lounge furniture that's older than I am. In the corner sits a keyboard and a drum kit flanked by three electric guitars and three small amps.

"This is Tony," one of my new friends says.

A gray-haired man explodes out of a pack of people, beaming, and begins pumping my hand like he's running for office. "Tony," he says. "Bob Solomon."

I recognize him immediately as one of the top reconstructive hand surgeons in the world. "Doctor Solomon, nice to meet you," I say. "I'm a big fan of yours."

"Thank you! Now, please, call me Bob."

"I'll try." He laughs. I wave my hand at the view. "This location is incredible."

"I know, right?" He leans in and whispers. "Tony, we found it, man."

I blink, confused, not sure what *it* is.

"Paradise." He waves his hand at the view. "I mean, look at this. We've figured it out. And nobody knows. You have to promise to keep it to yourself."

"So, wait, you live here...."

"And work a mile away. Have you heard of the Pink Palace?"

I have.

The Pink Palace. Legendary facility where Dr. Solomon and a few other internationally known plastic surgeons provide both cosmetic and reconstructive services for nearly the entire population of the Caribbean. He names his colleagues. I know them all. Well, I know of them. I've read their articles explaining some of the latest techniques in repair of hand injuries and skin cancers. They are bona fide superstars in the field of reconstructive surgery. Someone slaps a cold beer in my hand and Dr. Solomon leads me to his kitchen. He introduces me to two nurses who work with him at the Pink Palace. We clink bottles. We laugh. And then Dr. Solomon—Bob—claps me on the back.

"OK, he's here. Let's get started."

I blink and smile, once again confused.

He wags his head and I follow him into the living room. He nods at the instruments in the corner. "You play, right?"

"I do. I'm not great. In fact, full disclosure, I'm kind of a hack."

"A hack. Right. Migration."

"You heard of my band?" I am beyond shocked that these plastic surgery gods have heard of my rinky-dinky band. Sorry, my rinky-dinky *cover* band. I was under the impression that most of the people who see us play have never previously heard of us.

"Are you kidding? We vetted you. Now grab the 'caster in the middle. That's yours. For tonight."

He grins. I rest my beer bottle on one of the amps and strap on the electric guitar. I fiddle with it, get the feel of it, strum a couple of chords, trying to get the magic back in my fingers. Bob and one of the other doctors pick up guitars, a nurse sits behind the drum set, and another doc pulls a stool up to the keyboards. He plugs in and we tune up.

"So, here is the coolest moment of all time," Bob says. "One day I'm at work and I get a call that Keith Richards is on a yacht and he's injured his hand. I arrange to have a boat take me to him. It's really him. He looks like he's about two hundred years old and has been dead for a week. But it's Keith freaking Richards. He's cut his hand. Minor cut. I treat him. Couple of sutures. He's very gracious, wants to know if there's anything he can do to thank me. I say, 'Well, Keith, as a matter of fact...' and I invite him to the house. He comes over that night and, get this"—Bob pauses, a giddy grin spreading across his face—"Keith Richards *jams with us*."

"No way," I say.

"Way. Keith freaking Richards. Of the Rolling freaking Stones."

"He wasn't bad, for an old guy," one of the nurses says, and we all break up.

"So I got to cross that off my bucket list," Bob says. "Well, all right. You ready, Tony?"

"Yep. Fair warning. I'm not as good as Keith Richards."

The group cracks up again and we start to jam. At first we fool around, each of us taking a short solo, improvising, making noise, and then Bob signals us to stop for a second and he plays the introduction to "American Girl," by Tom Petty. I fake my way through without embarrassing myself too much. We finish that song and jump into another tune, "Uncle John's Band," by the Grateful Dead, and then another, and another. Then we rock our way into Santana's "Evil Ways." An attractive woman in a low-slung sarong, who'd been standing right in front of us, swaying to the music, her eyes closed, suddenly steps forward and starts singing, *"You've got to change your evil ways...baby!"* She's good. No. She's great. And we're all grooving to the song and the other players in the group are smiling and nodding, and I realize that I'm here, now, jamming with these three rock star plastic surgeons, people I've heard about and look up to, together, in the same band, holding my own.

Later, we take a break, gather in the kitchen, and drink flaming ouzo shots. When I say flaming, that's not a euphemism. These drinks are in fact on fire. I knock back two or three in a row, and then I'm playing again, ripping (OK, stumbling) through a solo. Then I'm sleeping it off, curled up on a soft couch overlooking the blue, blue water placid as a pool. Sometime after dawn, sober, exhausted, exhilarated, I wind my little SUV back down the treacherous hill, drive to the airport, and pick up Amy.

She takes one look at me and gives me her dubious, what-the-hell-have-you-got-yourself-into face. "You look like crap," she says as she slings her suitcase into the trunk of the SUV. "Tell me I'm not gonna regret this."

"You're gonna love it," I tell her. And she does, we both do. For the rest of the week my new friends join us at local restaurants and bars, entertain us at Bob's house, and lounge with us on beach chairs on the snow-white sand. For the first time in my life, I feel as if I've been inducted into a fraternity of inspiring, world-class peers, the fraternity I've always wanted to join.

And maybe—*just maybe*—I actually might belong.

12

Migration

"*Youner!*"

"Yep, it's me."

I picture Beverly Hills plastic surgeon Dr. Romeo Bouley on the other end of the phone, his six-foot-three-inch body thrown back into his ergonomic chair, his shock of white hair sculpted high on his head resembling a sand trap at Pebble Beach, his feet and shoes that cost more than my whole wardrobe up on his antique oak desk cluttered with figurines, first editions, and other ridiculously expensive tchotchkes, copies of *The Hollywood Reporter, Daily Variety,* and *Playboy* comingled with current prestigious medical journals, boxes of Cuban cigars, gold-plated letter openers, personally autographed 8″ x 10″s of gorgeous starlets, and empty Perrier bottles, all illuminated by lamps at each far corner shaped and painted like naked women. I spent a month shadowing him in my last year of medical school, and the experience blew my mind.

"How are you, Doctor Bouley?"

"Humping, bumping, trying to stay out of trouble and failing miserably."

"So, nothing's changed."

"*Hail* no. I'm still fooling 'em, baby. So, talk to me. You wanna come back to Beverly Hills to be my apprentice for a year after your residency, is that it? You just cannot stay away from the sunshine, starlets, and porn stars? Or is it just me and my dashing good looks?"

"I guess I'm completely transparent. And apparently shallow."

"Ha!" he roars. "OK, Youner, sell me. Give me your pitch to be my next fellow."

"My pitch?" I pause. "I don't really have a pitch. I just want to learn. I want to be the best. And in order to be the best, you have to work with and learn from the best. After five years of working with some amazing doctors here in Michigan, I have to say, you're the best I've ever seen. I'd love to spend a year learning from the master to finish up my education."

"If you think blowing smoke up my ass will get me to give you a fellowship position, you're absolutely right."

Now I laugh.

"You're sure there's nothing better out there for you?" he asks.

"I'm sure."

I decide not to tell him that I've been turned down for a job by all three of the major plastic surgery practices in the area.

I also don't tell him about the one offer I did get with a relative newcomer to the area, a plastic surgeon in Rockford. I shudder when I think about that one.

* * *

"What kind of practice do you have?" I ask the Rockford doc during our interview.

"What do you mean?" The doctor speaks in a quiet, lulling monotone. I imagine spending hours with him every day and needing to prop my eyelids open with toothpicks to stay awake.

"What type of patients do you see?" I ask.

"Oh. Well." He clears his throat, pauses, and finally whispers in his brain-numbing drone. "Here's a typical day. I begin early and drive to all the local jails."

"Jails?"

"Yes. I would say that the bulk of my practice consists of patients in jails and prisons."

"Prisons?" I hope he can't hear how loudly I gulp.

"That's what I said. Now, where was I? Oh, yes. Typical day. So, OK, normally, every morning, I drive to the jails and prisons and check out the different abscesses, boils, and injuries...."

"Wow, I actually know about prison care. I spent my psychiatry rotation in medical school at the Ionia maximum security prisons. The prisoners loved me. They nicknamed me Pretty Boy and told me that they were going home with me. Heh-heh." I get no response. I'm thinking, *Are you freaking kidding me?*

"Anyway, the good news is that we have an opening in the practice. I'm looking for someone to take responsibility for a number of prisons an hour away, while I do a little more cosmetic work. I think you would fit right in. We're a fun group. We have casual dress Fridays, a group get-together one Thursday a month at Olive Garden...."

I block out the rest. I mumble something about wanting to think about it and having to go. Then I immediately dial Dr. Romeo Bouley.

* * *

"Youner," Dr. Romeo Bouley says, and then repeats my nickname slowly, running it into three long lyrical syllables. *"You—nnn—errrrrr."*

The phone goes silent.

I know Dr. Bouley hasn't hung up because I hear the crackle of a match struck and the sucking down of expensive cigar smoke.

"When you were here a couple of years ago..."

"Five years ago, actually."

"Wow. OK. Five years ago. Back then I was doing very well. Right now? Through...the...*roof.* We're a rocket ship, Tony. The practice is exploding. I've hired two docs, guys you'll love, and I need to hire one more. Missing that one piece. I've interviewed half a dozen candidates, haven't found the right fit. Trying to figure out what to do. And then you call out of the blue. Like you are sent from the angels above. So you just might be that missing piece I need."

"Missing piece to do what?"

Dr. Bouley blows out a puff of smoke and then I hear his chair creak as I picture him lifting his legs off his desk, pulling up closer to the phone as he whispers, "To carry out my plan for global domination."

"Which is?"

"First, we're going to take over Beverly Hills. The four of us. Me, my two partners, and you. Then we conquer all of Los Angeles. Then the world. So, I guess I have to slam my one question right back at you." He pauses theatrically. "Are you in? Are you with us? Do you want to be a Master of the Universe?"

"I..."

"Yes?"

I think about Amy telling her parents that we'll come back to settle down in Michigan after my fellowship year. I can't lie.

"I can't promise."

An hour passes.

Or at least that's how long the thirty-second pause feels.

"I appreciate your honesty," Dr. Romeo Bouley says finally. "Before I can proceed, I must ask you to promise me one thing."

I swallow, scrunch my forehead. I'm pretty sure I shouldn't agree to anything, but I say, "OK..."

"Promise."

"I promise."

"Promise me that you'll be open. That if I hire you, you will consider the possibility that you will stay after your one-year fellowship is over."

"Yes. I will promise that."

"Then you're hired."

"I am?"

"Yes."

"Thank you. This is great. When do you want me to start?"

"Yesterday."

* * *

We scramble, somehow managing to leave for California within two weeks. Amy finds a position at Children's Hospital in Los Angeles. We cram all our furniture and winter clothes into a storage facility, pack my little dog, Theodore, the rest of our clothes, and all the essentials that will fit into my RAV4 and a U-Haul trailer. After tearful good-byes to Amy's parents, which we soften with promises that we will be back, we head West. On our way out of town, we stop to say good-bye to Duke, cofounder of the legendary (in our minds anyway) Migration. We hug, and Duke hands me several CDs he's made for our trip, "mixes for the road to match your every mood," he calls them. As I pop in the first one, I realize that of all the people I met after medical school, including our gang of five residents, the person I feel closest to is Duke.

Amy and I hit the open road for Hollywood, determined to live a brand-new adventure in uncharted territory, carefree, no regrets, unencumbered. Except for our $250,000 (yes, that's a quarter million dollars) of debt. "A year of fun in the sun" is how we see our time in LA. After which we vow to get serious and figure out exactly what we want to do when we grow up.

We find an apartment in Westwood near the UCLA campus. We buy Amy a reliable used car for her commute to work, which turns out to be a minimum of an hour each way, often in hellacious bumper-to-bumper traffic.

"Welcome to LA," she says, staggering into the apartment and collapsing onto the couch after her second day.

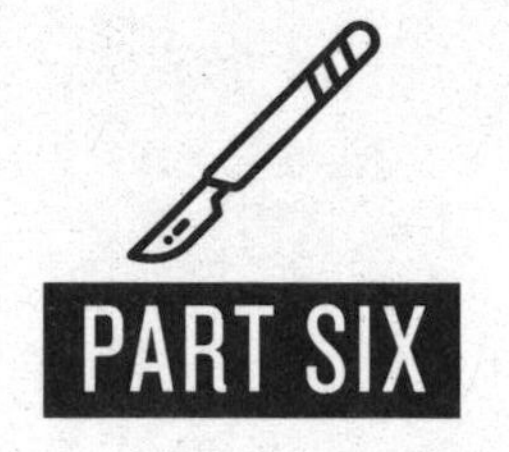

PART SIX

FELLOWSHIP—YEAR SIX

13

The Capital of Plastic Surgery

Beverly Hills. 90210. I pause for a moment in the hallway outside Dr. Romeo Bouley's office. Standing there, everything feels so vividly familiar: the stained-glass windows in the burnished oak doors opening into the office, the leather couches, abstract art, Oriental rugs, and the array of gaudy and strange naked lady lamps with their tatas positioned strategically throughout the waiting room. Carla, the receptionist, a former patient who came in for a nose job and apparently never left, greets me as I poke inside the waiting room. She is olive-skinned with dark hair flowing down to the middle of her back, a dancer's posture, an easy smile, and a clear lack of patience for incompetence. Carla runs the office with drill sergeant precision. We hit it off immediately.

Carla brings me back to Dr. Bouley, who leaps from his chair and embraces me like a prodigal son returning from a year at sea. He then grips me by the arm and introduces me to his partners, the team primed to take Hollywood, and apparently the world, by storm. First, I meet Dr. George, a tall, blond, WASPy, earnest, even-keeled kind of guy from Vermont who seems as out of place as maple syrup in an over-the-top sushi restaurant. Then I meet Dr. Bruce, short, thick-shouldered, thick-necked, built like a wrestler, black wavy hair, Persian, a hugger, opinionated, passionate, and occasionally hot-tempered. Carla, George, Bruce, and I form an instant and unlikely alliance. We will become as close as family.

Carla takes me to the reception area and lays out the typical workweek. Dr. Bouley operates every morning beginning at seven thirty and sees patients every afternoon. George and Bruce operate in the afternoons. Carla says that I will operate every morning with Dr. Bouley and whenever George or Bruce need me. The workday normally ends by seven. Most evenings, Carla, George, and Bruce eat at the Hamburger Hamlet downstairs, unwinding, decompressing, recapping the day, gossiping, and allowing the clogged arteries of LA traffic to ease. I don't mind the extra hour or so, since Amy has begun to moonlight at Kaiser Hospital two or three nights a week.

"Not a bad schedule," I say. "I'm used to working the graveyard shift."

"Well, it helps having the OR right here," Carla says. "Feels like we never leave. My boyfriend doesn't love that."

"What about Doctor George and Doctor Bruce? Are they married or do they have girlfriends?"

"Are you kidding? Who would have them?"

Carla winks so I know she's kidding.

I think.

* * *

It takes less than two weeks for me to feel part of Team Bouley. We just *click*. We work together seamlessly, a finely oiled machine, keeping on schedule, staying on track, operating on patients with epic precision and uncommon success. The office constantly buzzes, the waiting room, OR, and recovery room always bursting. We serve a specific clientele, the wealthy and prominent in business, and the Hollywood elite, the movers and shakers in film, TV, print, and porno. A far cry from the woolly wilds of Michigan.

When it comes to procedures, we're a one-stop shop. Nose jobs, neck lifts, facelifts, eye enhancement, breast augmentations and reductions, thigh work, tummy tucks, buttocks sculpting, liposuction. Dr. Romeo Bouley works tirelessly, effortlessly, brilliantly. He is a magician, a wizard, his knife is his wand. He's a savant with a scalpel. I learn a new technique every day. My confidence soars, my competence skies. All within the first *two weeks.*

The beginning of week three, a producer from a well-known TV cable network calls Dr. Bouley. He puts the producer on speaker so we can all hear. The producer says they are filming a piece at the Playboy Mansion and invites Dr. Bouley to be included.

"Oh, absolutely," he says, clamoring, as always, to bask in the spotlight. "Can I bring my colleagues with me?"

"You can bring one person," the producer says.

Dr. Bouley hangs up and grins, I believe, directly at me.

Suddenly, I revert to the horny, hopelessly virginal sixteen-year-old boy I was back in Michigan, where I fantasized about the models in *Playboy* magazine and longed to visit the famous mansion. Hugh Hefner lived the life—spending his days in silk pajamas surrounded by Playmates and Playboy Bunnies who tended to his every wish in the grotto, game room, and bedroom. I'd read all about the mansion and still couldn't get my head around the reality of it. I imagine entering a room with a waterbed for a floor, a bevy of half-naked beauties draped all over me, offering me cocktails, finger food, full-body massages....

"Choose me," I say to Dr. Bouley as if in a trance. "Please. I'm a loser from Michigan. I may never get this chance again."

"Oh, so you want to go to the mansion?"

"I do," I say. "I really do. My wife will understand. I want to go. I have to go. *Please.*"

He scratches his chin and then nods at Carla, George, and Bruce, who slowly, silently, reluctantly evacuate Dr. Bouley's office, closing the door behind them.

"I have a deal for you," Dr. Bouley says.

"Anything," I say.

"Commit to joining the practice. Sign the contract." He yanks open his desk drawer and fishes out a legal document. "I keep it right here. I've already filled in your name. All you have to do is sign. That's it. Done deal. And then you're a partner. As a signing bonus, I will take you to the Playboy Mansion. But you must sign now."

I stare at the contract. The sentences blur, swim in front of my eyes. I feel dizzy, as my hormonal adolescent dreams dance before me like sugar plum fairies in bikinis. I lean onto Dr. Bouley's desk to steady myself. I look up and search Dr. Bouley's eyes. He shows no expression. He pops a cigar into his mouth, and slowly slides the contract toward me.

"Simple, clean, painless," he says. "Sign."

"Can I...?" I stop. I start again. "What if I...?" I clear my throat. "How about this? I will promise to seriously consider it. Honest and truly. I will *seriously* consider it. Or maybe you can you give me an hour or two to figure it out?" I think about the fury I would face from Amy if I made this decision without her input. I picture weeks of being banished to sleep alone on the two-person love seat in our tiny apartment.

"So, that's a no."

"No. Yes. I mean, it's a...qualified no. But I'm adding serious consideration...."

Dr. Bouley is having none of it. He presses his intercom. "Carla, send in George." He turns to me. "Taking George might be a mistake. He'll see one Playmate and explode in his khakis. But I can't take Bruce. He'll go nuts, probably cannonball with his hairy back into the pool, and get us banned from the mansion for life."

"Maybe next time," I say, weakly.

"No next time," he says, with no room for equivocation. Clearly, no means no.

George pokes his head into the office. "Yes?"

"You like Bunnies, right?" Dr. Bouley says.

"Oh, yeah. Sure. I like puppies better."

"I'm talking about the kind at the Playboy Mansion."

"Oh," George's voice quivers. "*Ohhhhhhh.*"

Bruce shoves his head in next to George's. "You can't take him to the mansion. He's never seen a woman wearing less than three layers of clothing. He's from Vermont, for God sake. He's more comfortable with a moose than a Playboy Bunny."

"Oh, like Persia is the nudity capital of the Middle East," George says.

"This is all your fault," Dr. Bouley says to me.

"He still won't commit?" George says.

Dr. Bouley says no, wags his cigar toward George. "I'm taking you. Go home and take a series of increasingly cold showers. Maybe rub one out. We leave tomorrow right after Youner and I do that breast augment."

"Maybe it's better to maintain the fantasy," I say. Even I don't believe it.

George, Bruce, and Dr. Bouley all shake their heads.

The next morning Dr. Bouley and I prepare for a breast enlargement on Gina, a gorgeous Italian model. The operation goes smoothly, without any complications. At one point, Dr. Bouley lowers his voice and says to me, "I wasn't going to do this, but I'm offering you a second chance. If you sign the contract right now, I'll take you instead of George, who you can hear panting on the other side of this wall."

"I'll consider it, *really* consider it...."

"Oh, stop it. Let's finish her up. I don't want to keep Hef waiting."

We finish the procedure, give Gina plenty of time in recovery, and then discharge her. I watch as Dr. Bouley and George head out for their dream trip to the Playboy Mansion. With the heaviest of hearts, I look at Carla.

"Poor baby," she says, rolling her eyes.

In the early evening, around six thirty, as Carla shuts down business for the day, a call comes through for me. Gina. She has a complication. She's bleeding profusely. I tell her to meet me at the office ASAP. I call Dr. Bouley on his cell at the mansion. "Doctor Bouley, we have to bring Gina back to surgery. There's a complication. She's bleeding."

He seems surprised. "She was fine. Well, these things happen. That's OK. I've had enough of this place, anyway. I'll tell George to call a cab. If I can find him."

My heart sinks. "Is he having a good time?"

"Oh, Youner. Life changer. Lost him somewhere around the grotto. He will never be the same. And to think, it could've been you."

* * *

A couple of hours later, we complete what amounts to a second procedure on Gina, the gorgeous Italian model. We drain out the excess blood, restore and resuture the work we'd previously done, and after we're sure everything is fine, we send her home. As we change out of our scrubs, Dr. Bouley says, with a hint of nostalgia and regret, "You really didn't miss much. I was just messing with you. The mansion's seen better days."

"Are you just saying that to make me feel better?"

"No, actually, I'm not. It's run-down. Needs a major upgrade."

"Really? What about the grotto?"

"A mess. Pigeon and geese shit all over. Unidentified floaters in the pool. Muck on the bottom. It looked like it hadn't been dredged since the seventies. Animals everywhere. Wandering around. Crapping, pissing, stinking, out of control. Horrible."

"What about the women?"

"I saw a few models when we were setting up for the interview. They have been touched up big time for the magazine. Photoshop City. I'll be honest. Gina is way hotter than anyone I saw there."

"Seriously?"

"Seriously." He takes a beat. "I'm glad you didn't sign that contract."

"Sounds like I would've felt ripped off."

"Oh, definitely, and..." He lays a hand on my shoulder. "I don't want to bribe you. You should sign the contract only if you really want to be here."

Just one of the reasons I like and admire Dr. Bouley.

Still. A wave of sadness washes up on my shores as I realize I missed my one and only shot at the Playboy Mansion.

The Playboy freaking Mansion!

* * *

The next day, Gina calls the office. She's bleeding again. This time we arrange to admit her to UCLA Medical Center. I have no privileges at the hospital, but after my day at work, I visit Gina to see how she's doing. She's showing major improvement. The doctors there have treated her and as a precaution want to keep her overnight. I hang out with her in her room. She thanks me for coming, knowing I didn't have to. She asks how I'm adjusting to life in LA. I shake my head. It's a lot different than Michigan, I tell her. The people, the pace, the lifestyle. Sometimes I feel like Dorothy, looking around wide-eyed, going, *I don't think we're in Kansas anymore*.

"I know," Gina says, and tells me to take advantage of my time here. We talk like a couple of old friends. We laugh about my pale, ghostlike complexion, and she tells me I have to put in some serious beach time. She suggests I take in the Hollywood nightlife too. When I tell her Amy and I like to dance, she recommends a couple of trendy clubs. I come back the next day, a Saturday, and sit with her. She tells me how much she appreciates the time I'm spending with her, reiterates that she knows it's my day off and I don't have to do this, appreciates so much that I'm going beyond the call of duty. When I leave, she says, "Tony, thanks for taking such good care of me."

After the doctors discharge Gina from UCLA, Dr. Bouley and I set up regular appointments at the office to monitor her. She comes in every other week for a couple of months. Although she's not technically my patient, I continue to check in on her. She always seems pleased to see me. We joke around and she asks if I ever made it to the dance clubs she suggested. When I say not yet, she tells me to be sure to mention her name when I do.

One Saturday, a week or so after Gina's last appointment, a loud knock at our apartment door jars me. I open the door and find our mail carrier standing outside. He hands me what looks like an innocuous envelope.

"Got a certified letter for you," he says.

I sign for it, go back inside the apartment, and open the envelope, expecting some cute thank-you card an Italian model sends you after you take awesome care of her. Looking back, I can't believe what a naïve fool I was.

I ease out a letter.

It's from an attorney.

Gina, the beautiful Italian model, who thanked me for taking such good care of her, who offered suggestions for clubs and restaurants as if she were my friend, is threatening to sue me.

In her attorney's letter, she accuses me of patient abandonment, improper treatment, lying about my medical background, not being forthright about my skills, of having a history of malpractice....

The complaints continue, but the words blur into an inky mess.

I do manage to read one sentence, underlined and written in bold at the bottom of the page.

Her attorney writes that if I do not pay Gina $100,000, she will proceed with the lawsuit and sue me for a lot more than that.

Welcome to Beverly Hills.

I feel like throwing up. I fold the letter and sit down. I feel a stabbing pain in the pit of my stomach. Within seconds, I begin going through Elisabeth Kübler-Ross's Five Stages of Grief.

First, denial.

This can't be happening.

Gina and I were friends. Or, at least, friendly. I went above and beyond the call of duty for her. She thanked me for looking after her. She seemed genuinely appreciative. This has got to be a mistake. I thought we were freaking *friends.*

Stage two arrives.

Anger.

That *bitch*!

For one thing, she's rich. She's a wildly successful model who lives in Beverly Hills, and she's suing *me*? I start pacing through my crappy little hovel of an apartment: $250,000 in debt, with a wife who's working two jobs, and this rich socialite is trying to extort money out of me, money I not only don't have now, but will likely never have.

I'm not sure which stages of grief follow, because the anger stage grips my heart like a clamp and twists my brain like a cyclone. I call Dr. Bouley at home and, with my words stumbling all over each other, tell him about the letter.

"What? She's threatening to sue you? What a nut job."

"I'm sick to my stomach," I say.

"Don't worry. I've got the best lawyers in the city. We'll get you out of this. This bullshit will never see the light of day, I promise you. Take a couple of deep breaths, pour yourself a scotch. Or go for a run. Rub one out. Do whatever you need to do to calm down. This is all gonna go away. I promise you."

"It's just that I've never been sued before."

"Yeah, well, you're young."

"I'm *young.* What does that mean?"

"This line of work? These patients? You get sued every other year. Goes with the territory. Nature of the business."

"You get sued *every other year*?"

"Oh, yeah. At least. Now don't worry about this. I'm on it."

He hangs up. I wrap my arms around my middle and collapse in a shriveled heap onto the couch. My forehead feels warm and clammy.

And, of course, I think of my dad.

Is this how he felt?

Horribly betrayed and scared to death?

I understand, intellectually, that there are worse things that can happen to someone. I try putting things in perspective. I think about my job, my family, my Amy.

How did my dad get through nearly a year of this?

Of course, he didn't. He lost a piece of himself when he got sued. And he never really recovered.

Is this how I want to live, knowing that any patient, at any time, can go bonkers and sue me, can try to ruin me, even when I've done absolutely nothing wrong? In this case, even went out of my way to be the doctor I want to be? How did it backfire so horribly?

Is this the career I want?

Is this the life I want?

Yes. It is.

I know it is.

I know too that I will have to learn to accept this part of it, to learn to live with a constant undercurrent of uncertainty and even fear.

Over the next few days, I experience all five of Kübler-Ross's stages of grief, though not necessarily in order, and not always separately. I stay in a state of anger for only a short time, a day maybe, and then depression settles in, debilitating me. During this time, I experience a minor need to bargain. So I ask God, "If you take this ridiculous lawsuit away, I promise I will..."

The problem is I don't even know what to promise. Do I promise to be kinder to everyone, a better husband, a better son, a better coworker, a better doctor? Do I promise to go to church more often? I do mumble that promise, but the bargaining stage of grief quickly falls away, and with Dr. Bouley's assurances reverberating through my brain, I land heavily into the fifth stage: acceptance.

"I can't fight this," I tell myself, "but from now on I'll be prepared. I'll still expect the best of my patients, but I'll always be ready mentally in case this happens again. I need to expect that someday it will."

One day, after months of hanging over me like the blade of an invisible guillotine, the attempt to legally extort me goes away. My malpractice attorney informs me that Gina has withdrawn her threat of a lawsuit.

"I told you not to worry," Dr. Bouley says to me. "Although I know that's easier said than done."

"I am so relieved," I say. "I feel like I can breathe again."

"Well, I admit, I didn't see it coming, not from her."

"She was so nice. So appreciative."

"Those are the worst. The ones who suck you in and then blindside you."

"You said you get sued every other year?"

Dr. Romeo Bouley shrugs. "At least." And then he adds, with a wink, "Small price to pay."

14

Business as Usual in La La Land

I'm pulling a reverse Beverly Hillbillies. I'm going to go from the swimming pools and movie stars of Beverly Hills back to the backwoods boonies of Michigan. It's become increasingly clear that after I fulfill my commitment to stay in Beverly Hills for a year, I can't stay beyond that. At our weekly dinners out at low-end restaurants we can barely afford, Amy and I try to imagine settling here, raising a family. But when we start telling stories of the Hollywood glitterati we meet and their spouses, our parents burst out of us (especially from me), each story ending with one of the same two punch lines: "Bouley's is all about the money" or "Beverly Hills is not the place for us to raise a family."

As the months pass and the glamour fades, we feel a longing to return to our roots. We both know it: when the year ends, I'll have to tell Dr. Bouley that I can't sign a contract and we'll go back to Michigan. For now, though, we'll enjoy the year-round sunshine and the bizarre world of Hollywood plastic surgery—its state of mind—that feels foreign to us in so many ways.

Each day at Dr. Bouley's brings me an entirely different experience, ranging from inspiring to cringeworthy. Although I'm learning more about cosmetic surgery in this past year than I have in the previous five, the sum total of my experiences confirms to me that being a Beverly Hills plastic surgeon just isn't the right fit for me.

* * *

This week's stranger than fiction case.

An adult film actress.

I am, I admit, familiar with her "body of work."

Having turned the corner on thirty, perhaps even reaching thirty-five, she schedules a consultation. She has a concern. When screening her most recent film, she thought she looked too gaunt.

"I think I'm getting too harsh looking," she says, frowning. "What do you guys think?" I mumble something about not really paying much attention to her face, but she presses on.

"I want three things," she says. "First, I want to look younger."

"Not a problem," Dr. Bouley says. "We will take some fat from your butt, a small amount, and inject that into your face."

"OK," she says and then cups her breasts. "These. I need to go up a size."

"Easy," Dr. Bouley says.

"And number three," she says, "I want to bleach my backside."

Both Dr. Bouley and I blink rapidly. He breaks our stunned silence. "Let me understand this. You want to bleach your..."

"My butthole. I want to turn it white."

"I'm going to have to say no to that," Dr. Bouley says. "I'm not familiar with that procedure. Never done it."

"It's for my work." She pouts. "Other girls are doing it."

"Well, you should get a referral because I'm going to pass on that one."

"I'm doing it for my career...."

"I get that," Dr. Bouley says. He looks at me.

"I get it too?" I say.

"So, we'll have to pass on the dye job," Dr. Bouley says.

"Fine. We'll do the other two." She scrunches her face. "Make me look like Reese Witherspoon."

"From the neck up," Dr. Bouley mutters.

* * *

I see a woman, midforties, a pretty Midwestern girl-next-door type, who seems, at first, to be kind of, well, *normal.* She comes in for a consultation about some liposuction and breast implants—nothing crazy, nothing extreme—and our conversation flows, pleasantly, easily. After my experience with Gina the Italian model, alarm bells routinely clang inside my head, but I can't stop thinking, *Wow, with all the unusual personalities who come in and out of this place, this woman seems pretty straightforward and low key, like the people back home.* We schedule her procedures, she thanks me, and I look forward to seeing her again. A couple weeks later, as we're about to begin her surgery, I ask, casually, "So, what do you do for a living?"

She smiles demurely. "Well, two things. First, I'm a hand and foot model."

"Oh," I say. "Nice."

I can see that. Her hands and feet look relatively photogenic. I could picture myself flipping through a magazine and seeing her hand holding a container of yogurt or her foot slipping into an athletic shoe.

"I do pretty well," she says, "but that's not how I make the big money."

"Oh?"

"Yeah. I make my living—a really good living—off of the internet. I buy and sell stuff on eBay."

I perk up. "That's really interesting. I used to be addicted to eBay. I spent hours and hours buying and selling old comic books, ones I always wanted when I was a little kid. I still have them. It's so cool that you do that. What do you buy and sell?"

"Used women's underwear," she says.

"Used...Oh...I never..."

I stall, trying to figure out how to end that sentence.

"I go to flea markets and buy used panties, bras, thongs, whatever, seal them in a plastic bag, and sell them to horny guys online. I make a fortune."

"That is so..." A long list of words scrolls through my head, including but not limited to: *Nasty. Revolting. Disgusting. Unhygienic. Stinky.* Fortunately, the word "enterprising" slides out of my mouth.

"The more used the better," she says, winking, and then laughing.

I laugh too loudly, faking it, feeling just a tiny bit creeped out.

The things we do to make a living.

* * *

And then I witness and, sadly, am party to, incidents that I find truly disturbing. Two of these occur toward the end of my one-year fellowship with Dr. Bouley. They contribute to Amy and me leaving Beverly Hills and returning to Michigan.

Occasionally, Dr. Bouley allows other surgeons to use his operating room. In retrospect, I'm sure he rented them the space. More than once, Dr. Bouley assigns me to assist one plastic surgeon in particular. Let's call him Dr. X.

Dr. X brings in a patient, a very large African American woman who wants liposuction. After the anesthesiologist knocks her out, Dr. X and I each tackle a thigh. We work side by side, in silence. About two and a half hours into the procedure, after taking off a couple of liters of fat, Dr. X swipes his sweaty forehead and announces, "That's it. We're done."

I look at the time and the patient. "I think we can take some more off. She could look a lot better."

"Yeah, well, we're going to stop," Dr. X says.

"Are you sure?"

"Look, I gave her a special deal. I knocked a couple thousand off my price. She's got HIV anyway, so let's just quit."

I'm beyond troubled by Dr. X's lack of ethics. Just because this patient received a discount doesn't mean that she should get a less-than-optimal outcome. And what does her HIV status have to do with any of this? He's actually using the fact that she's HIV-positive to rationalize ending the operation early and giving her a lesser result.

I'm also deeply concerned that he is turning me into his accomplice, assuming I would understand and agree with his decision. I decide to tell Dr. George, Dr. Bruce, and Carla about Dr. X during one of our afterwork happy hour sessions.

"You're getting worked up," Dr. George says after I finish the story.

"Well, yeah," I protest. "It's outrageous."

"It is," Dr. Bruce says, catching Carla's eye. "And it's..."

She finishes his sentence. "Business as usual."

"Maybe he was just being cautious," I say. "Maybe he thought a longer surgery would be riskier for her."

"Yeah, maybe," Dr. George says. "That must've been it."

Our table goes silent. For several seconds the only sound is Carla stirring the ice cubes in her glass.

"Business as usual," she repeats. "And you know it."

* * *

A month or so later, I again assist Dr. X with a liposuction surgery. This time he approaches the procedure with the recklessness of Kobayashi sucking up hot dogs.

The FDA recommends that doctors remove a maximum of five liters of fat from a patient during liposuction. Beyond that, we are supposed to admit the patient to a hospital overnight where transfusions are available if needed. I'm acutely aware of this since our operating room is on the tenth floor of an office building, several miles away from the nearest hospital.

We begin liposuction on an extremely obese woman. Dr. X has specifically requested me to assist. He's told Dr. Bouley that he's comfortable with me. I want to say I'm flattered, but after our last liposuction on the patient with HIV, I feel highly skeptical. I want to finish this procedure and then tell Dr. Bouley that I'd rather not work with Dr. X again.

We begin the liposuction. We hit one liter. We get to two liters. We hit three liters...four liters...five liters.

I assume we will now stop.

Dr. X keeps going.

I start to say something.

He waves me off.

We hit six liters.

Seven liters...eight liters...nine liters...ten liters...

At eleven liters, I say, as if he doesn't know, "We're at eleven liters."

"So?"

"I think we should stop. We're moving so much fat and so much blood..."

"It'll be fine. Let's keep going."

"I really think we should stop."

Dr. X rolls his eyes. "What are you worried about?"

"This isn't safe."

Dr. X shakes his head and snickers. "We're gonna keep going."

"Maybe you are, but I'm not."

He stares at me with undisguised disdain.

"I'm done," I say. "I'm not doing this anymore."

"Are you walking out on me?"

"Yes."

I snap off my gloves, remove my mask, and rip off my gown.

"Note my exit on the chart," I say. "I don't want anything to do with this."

"Fine. Have it your way. Wimp."

I storm out of the operating room. The door slams shut behind me. The moment I'm out of the operating room my breathing quickens, my head whirls, and my hands start to shake. I don't know what I should do. I could tell Dr. Bouley, but I doubt he'll care. He has essentially washed his hands of Dr. X and anything that happens in there. And I can hear Dr. George, Dr. Bruce, and Carla telling me over drinks that this is business as usual.

I feel faint. I find a chair and sit down.

The next day when I get back into the office I learn that Dr. X removed fourteen liters of fat from the patient.

I tell Amy the story.

"Why did he keep going? It was totally reckless."

"It was his attitude," I say. "He had this macho surgeon mentality thing going on. This ridiculous, condescending, downright dangerous swagger. 'I know what I'm doing. I'm in charge. Nothing can go possibly wrong.'"

"Like he knows everything," Amy says.

I shake my head in disgust. "As if he were playing God."

* * *

They say it ain't all about the money. But of course, in Beverly Hills, it is. We exist in the la-la world of cosmetic surgery filled with filthy rich people who will pay anything to find the fountain of youth. But what drives the practice beyond even the money is the competition. It seems like a cosmetic surgery rat race. Sadly, as Lily Tomlin once said, the trouble with the rat race is that even if you win, you're still a rat.

"The competition, that's what it's really about," Carla says to us over our end-of-the-day drinks. "If we say no to a particular procedure, we're only hurting ourselves because we know that somebody else will do it."

"So we might as well be the ones," Dr. George says.

"Plus, I honestly believe we will do a better job than Dr. Schmoe Joe down the block. We're better than our competition," Dr. Bruce says.

"That's Joe Schmoe, but close enough," Carla says.

"I was not born in your country," Dr. Bruce says.

"It's such a different demographic here," I say, not looking up, expecting to see a sea of eye rolling, lost in my own conversation. "For example, I can't get over the number of people who get liposuction. It's not always the best alternative."

Everybody's gone past eye rolling. They're into staring at me like I'm either an idiot or hippy socialist. Or possibly both. I don't care. I keep going. I'm venting.

"You know what? I might even try to talk a patient out of liposuction. I really would. I would absolutely say, 'Why don't you hire a trainer, work with a dietician, put down the Cinnabon, and eat a freaking salad, try to lose some weight the old-fashioned way? That would be my recommendation.'"

After a long horrified silence, Dr. Bruce says, "Seriously?"

"Seriously."

"There's no money in that," Dr. George says. "And you're in the business of making money, especially if you work at Bouley's."

"No," I say, louder than I should, but not as strongly as I feel. "I'm not. I'm in a different business. I'm in the business of being a doctor."

* * *

Beyond the Beverly Hills plastic surgery culture—the gaudy taste, a doctor's office decorated with naked lady lamps, the sometimes questionable ethics and emphasis on commerce over cosmetics, profit over patients, and, yes, the *money, money, money*—I cannot put a price on what Dr. Romeo Bouley himself teaches me. In the field of plastic surgery, he is a visionary, a pioneer. He teaches me how to perform procedures I'd never even heard about. He shows me how to flip a patient's permanent frown into a smile. He's the first to show me how to optimally lift a neck. He shows me how to put in breast implants through an armpit. He teaches me how to inject fat and stem cells into the face.

And he shows me how to look at a face in three dimensions, rather than two.

"People think in terms of tightening and lifting," he says. "I see it a different way. It's really about volume, how a face is filled out, and determining how a face ages. You have to think in terms of drawing on paper versus sculpting with clay. Painting versus sculpting. I sculpt."

He's a plastic surgeon Michelangelo, Alexander Calder, and Bones McCoy from *Star Trek* all rolled into one.

I see his approach as revolutionary and profound.

As a young plastic surgeon, he changed my life.

* * *

Amy and I see the end and we vow to have fun before we leave.

While surfing the internet one day, I come across an ad looking for extras and dancers for *Dick Clark's New Year's Rockin' Eve*, which is being filmed in a week. This doesn't seem right because it's early November. I double-check. Yep. They're looking for dancers for New Year's Eve...*in November.* When it's 85 degrees in LA.

The company asks for some basic information and a picture. I find a nice photograph from our wedding. Feeling this is all a lark anyway, I send it in.

I get a return email inviting us to come to a studio in Hollywood for the event and telling us to be dressed to *party*. We're excited. We've made the cut! Hollywood is calling!

Amy and I dress for a New Year's Eve party. I wear a button-down shirt and khaki pants and Amy wears a dress. We arrive at the studio, find the stage entrance, and enter into a loud herd of wannabe New Year's Eve dancers. We're shocked. One group of older people wears suits and ties and granny dresses. A second group, younger, dresses in ratty clothes that look as if they were just pulled out of a dumpster, or cut-offs, torn jeans, stained and ripped T-shirts with skulls or wildly inappropriate sayings. It takes a twentysomething producer's assistant approximately two seconds to pull us out of the crowd.

She escorts us through a huge metal door that looks like it belongs on a vault. It leads down a dark hall to a soundstage. We join a dozen or so other couples. The assistant arranges us according to height or looks or...I'm not really sure what, then she disappears. A band appears on stage, a group we've never heard of, and then a voice comes over a PA system and booms, "OK, everybody...start dancing!" The band plays and we dance for about fifteen minutes. The band stops and the same voice comes over the PA system and booms, "That was great! Now we're gonna do the countdown! Pretend it's New Year's Eve, so count down with us and then scream and cheer and make a ton of noise. Ready? *Act.*"

And we do, counting down to the New Year in November, hollering, "Happy New Year!" We hug each other and hold a long kiss. Then the band starts playing again and we dance some more. After an hour, that band makes way for another band, then that band steps aside for a third band.

Amy leans over and shouts in my ear, "My feet are killing me!"

I scream back at her, "I operated for six hours today. My back is in spasm!"

We look longingly at the hallway leading to that metal door, a football field away, and I say to her, "We're prisoners. They're never gonna let us leave. We're trapped in here forever. We'll be forced to dance until we die. I'm not kidding. People have *died* during dance marathons."

Amy grimaces, leans on me, and says, "We have to get out of here."

"How?"

"We have only one choice."

I understand immediately, in a way that only someone who's been part of a two-doctor couple for years can. "No," I say. "We can't do that."

"We have to. It's the only way."

"But we agreed...."

"I know what we agreed," she says. "Screw it. Do it."

I look at her long and hard, my mind clicking through any other option I can think of.

I can think of none.

"OK," I say finally. "But just this once and never again."

"Absolutely. Never again."

And so I play the doctor card.

* * *

The band finishes playing a song, segues into their next number. Amy and I jog off the dance floor and find our stuff, balled up in a corner. I pull out my pager. I look for the producer's assistant, which is not hard, because she's twenty feet away, glaring at me like a prison guard preventing a jailbreak. I wave my pager and approach her.

"Hey, listen, I'm a doctor, and I'm getting paged."

She lowers her chin and makes what I'm pretty sure is her you-are-so–lying face.

So I rev it up.

"Yeah, I'm really sorry, but I have to go to the hospital to perform an, um, emergency abdominorhinomastopexy on a patient."

Another chin tilt. "Are you sure? What's the problem?"

"Yes, oh, yes, very sure, it's really serious. There's all this skin and guts and pus and stuff. Yes, super serious. He is going to die without an abdominorhinomastopexy. I have to go...*now*."

She still doesn't look convinced, but she caves. "Well, I don't suppose you carry like a doctor card or anything. Oh, never mind, if you have to go, go."

"Yeah. I do. Gotta go, gotta run. Really sorry. Happy New Year."

I grab Amy's hand and we bolt the hell out of there.

I've never been that happy to escape a New Year's Eve celebration in November when it's 85 degrees.

A month and a half later, on the real New Year's Eve, Amy and I barhop through Hollywood, each place more packed and depressing than the last. At eleven o'clock, we head back to our small apartment in Westwood, pop some champagne, pour a couple of glasses, snuggle on the couch with our dog, Theodore, tune in to *Dick Clark's New Year's Rockin' Eve,* and toast in the New Year in the most surrealistic way ever: watching ourselves dance on TV.

15

Say Goodbye to Hollywood

Several months before the end of my fellowship with Dr. Romeo Bouley, knowing that I am going to leave Beverly Hills and settle back in Michigan, I do what I do best: I research and I prepare.

Amy and I want to live near her parents, so I eliminate places like Grand Rapids and focus on the Detroit suburbs. Then I try to turn from medical doctor into spin doctor, crafting a letter of introduction that I'll send to plastic surgeons in the area, finessing what I fear are meager credentials into something so impressive that they'll consider hiring me to join their practice. I spend hours working on this letter until I feel it's perfect. Finally, satisfied, I send the letter to thirty-three plastic surgeons.

I receive two replies.

The first reply comes from a plastic surgeon I'll call Dr. Wacko. He sends me back an extremely enthusiastic response, inviting me to meet him at his office for an interview.

The second reply is from a Dr. Paneer. It seems slightly guarded, but he does mention in his letter that he might have a "lucrative opportunity for the right person."

I buy a conservative business suit from Men's Wearhouse for the two interviews, arrange to take off two days, and fly to Michigan. I get lost in the Detroit suburbs looking for Dr. Wacko's office, which he calls a surgery center. I actually drive past his office twice because it doesn't dawn on me that the cluster of dingy little office buildings in the crappiest part of town could possibly qualify as a surgery center. I figure I've taken a wrong turn and ended up in the projects. I double- and triple-check the address until sadly I realize that I have indeed come to Dr. Wacko's office. I park my rental car outside a rickety building with peeling cream-colored paint, a rusted rain gutter dangling dangerously over the front door. I look down at my new suit. I realize I'm seriously overdressed.

I take a seat in a chilly waiting room until finally, after a good (actually, truth be told, *bad*) twenty minutes of imagining what a catastrophic downward slide this will be from Beverly Hills, Dr. Wacko, a disheveled guy in his sixties, still in his scrubs, slouches out of a back area.

"Just finishing up," he says, shaking my hand. "Come on back, Tony. Let's talk. Beverly Hills, huh?"

"Yes."

"Great," he mutters, in a tone that clearly implies "Big freaking deal."

I follow him into his cramped, dark office. He pulls up a dusty torn window shade, revealing a window overlooking a landfill. He takes a seat on a creaky chair behind a desk piled with paperwork. I settle into a straight-backed chair across from him.

"So," he says. "What are you thinking?"

I rustle uncomfortably, fold my hands. I don't tell him that I'd prefer gouging my eyes out with a rusty scalpel than working here. Instead I say, "Well, I'm thinking about moving back to town, you know, to the area, and I was wondering if you might be interested in taking on a younger plastic surgeon. I'm not proud and I'll do whatever it takes, anything you need. I'll take your calls for you.

I'll help with your patients. Anything. Just to get started." When I feel I can grovel no more, I stop. He says nothing for at least thirty seconds.

"I'd like to ask you a question," he says at last.

"Sure."

"If you do a breast augmentation on a patient and she develops excess scar tissue—not your fault, it just happens—what would you do?"

I fidget before I answer. "I would do the surgery again."

"Would you charge her?"

Suddenly my forehead has a mind of its own, and I feel it furrowing without my consent. I repeat his question. "Would I charge her?" I take a moment and say, "I'd probably give her my time for free, but because I don't own an operating room, I can't pay for that, so I'm not sure how I would..."

"Oh, so you'd up-charge her implants to make some money off of that. I see. Next question."

"I didn't say..."

"*Next* question. Say you operate on a patient and she has a bleeding complication. What would you do?"

"I would get her to go to the hospital immediately. I'd meet her there, take care of her surgically if I needed to, and, of course, drain out all the blood...."

"Would you bill her insurance? And if her insurance didn't pay, would you charge her out of pocket and jack up the fee a little so you could make a little money? What would you do?"

I stiffen in my chair. Suddenly I feel like I'm on one of those horrible talk shows, and the guest thinks they're in for a nice surprise but gets blindsided by a screaming woman claiming he got her, her mom, and her daughter pregnant.

"I'm not sure where you're going with all this...."

Dr. Wacko smirks, then suddenly stands up and nearly throws himself across the desk until he's practically in my face. "What's the muscle that's right underneath the pectoralis major? Can you tell me what that is? Can you? *Huh?*"

I stammer. "No offense, but is there something wrong with you? Are you hypoglycemic? Do you need some orange juice?"

He eases back in his creaky chair and drums his fingers on his desk. "Look, this is very simple. This town isn't big enough for both of us."

"Excuse me?"

"This is a small town. You should go down to Detroit. Check out Grosse Pointe. That's the hot place. You seem like a nice young man so if you find something down there, feel free to call me for a reference. I got to do some surgery."

He stands, lowers his head so far it nearly disappears inside his scrubs, and charges out of the room. I'm left crouched in midair in his office, my hand extended ridiculously, expecting a farewell handshake that's clearly never coming.

Two minutes later, I slide into my rental car and, feeling more numb than upset, I call a friend in Grand Rapids who knows about my meeting with Dr. Wacko.

"How did it go?"

"He's in*sane*, I'm talking cuckoo crazy!" I say and tell him about my "interview."

When I finish, my friend says, "He's actually not nuts. He's diabolical. He has an agenda. He was trying to trip you up so that if you do decide to settle there he'd rat you out."

"Rat me out? How?"

"He'd tell the hospital he works at that he interviewed you and that he has a problem with your ethical standards."

"He was trying to entrap me?"

"Well, first he was trying to scare you away. Then, yeah, I'd call it entrapment. False accusation. Whatever. My advice? Do not go anywhere near that guy."

"Thanks," I say. "I'm crossing him off. I'm glad he's not my only hope." *Fine,* I think. *Better to find out about Doctor Wacko now. Besides, I'm only zero for one. I have a second, stronger lead.*

I hope.

* * *

The next day I travel to another suburb to meet Dr. Paneer at his office in a modern medical building a block away from the local hospital. I enter his waiting room. His receptionist greets me like an old friend, offers me coffee, tea, or water and a broad smile. Within minutes Dr. Paneer, a gushy guy in his early fifties is pumping my hand like he's actually happy to see me.

"Very nice of you to come all the way from California," he says. "Let me give you the grand tour." He leads me through two large, clean, well-appointed operating rooms. Dr. Paneer is calm, even deferential, and curious about me. The anti-Dr. Wacko.

"So, do you want to raise a family here?"

"Yes. That's the plan. Eventually."

"Well, this is a great community. Very family oriented. Oh." Standing in the doorway of one of his operating rooms, he gestures like Vanna White pointing out the grand prize. "This is Medicare approved so you can get insurance payments if you work out of here. And by the way, I own the building."

"That's a plus," I say, more impressed by the second.

"Oh, yes. *So.*" Dr. Paneer wags his head and hitches up his pants. He reminds me of a car salesman going in for the sale. "I would love to have you here."

"That's very nice," I say. Because it actually *does* seem very nice.

"I would love to have you join *our* family," he says, grinning now.

I look hard, but I see no downside. So I simply say, "That sounds great." Then I reach out to shake his hand.

Dr. Paneer grips my hand and widens his grin. "Wonderful. So you'll rent the space?"

My handshake deflates, goes limp as a rag. "Excuse me?"

"I'm excited to have you rent my operating room," he says.

"I don't want to rent anything. I thought you were interested in taking me in as a partner. In your practice. Kind of help me get started. Work together. That's what I wrote in my letter."

"Oh, no, I don't want any partners. I want a tenant. I have this great space. I thought you'd want to rent from me."

"*No!*" I say too loudly. "I didn't come all the way from California to check out operating room rentals. I'm a plastic surgeon. I want to join a practice."

"That's too bad," he says. "I probably should've read your letter more carefully instead of skimming." He shrugs and starts pumping my hand again. "Very nice meeting you."

There goes my new "family."

Make that zero for two.

* * *

With six weeks to go, I finalize the end of my fellowship with Dr. Bouley in his office one day after work, the only light coming from the glow of his numerous naked lady lamps. I tell him that I've made a truly difficult decision and that I will be moving back to Michigan. It's official. A done deal.

"I know you've been saying this right along, at least hinting at it since day one, but I'm still shocked." He rakes his fingers through the twin silver sand dunes of his hair. "I thought for sure you'd cave. Are you positive? You're really going to leave me?"

"Believe me, it was a tough decision," I say. "But, yeah, we're going back home."

"You know you're the first person who's ever turned me down."

"I guess I have a knack for being...different," I say, with a small laugh. "I'll probably regret it." The laugh dissolves.

"In all seriousness, if you change your mind, or if you get back to Michigan and it's not working out for whatever reason, you always have a place here."

"Thank you. That means a lot."

We stand. I reach out my hand. Dr. Romeo Bouley brushes it away and throws his arms around me. We hug. And not the Hollywood kind, where you're looking behind the person's back for someone better to hug. No, this is a true hug that means something.

A week later, after putting a deposit down on an apartment, Amy and I stand in the parking lot of an office building in Rochester, Michigan, an upscale suburb of Detroit that we will soon call home. We stare at the window of the first-floor suite that a contractor will build out into my office. At the moment, the panes in the window before me shimmering and blurring, I feel disoriented and numb. I have just signed a five-year lease. I will pay $6,000 a month.

Six thousand dollars. A month.

Every time I think of this my gonads shrivel up.

"I love it here," I say, trying desperately to believe it.

"Oh, yeah, it's great. Rochester is great," Amy says, sounding not entirely convinced.

"Giving up Beverly Hills, job security, celebrities, year-round sunshine..."

"Absolutely the right thing to do."

"Definitely. Not a doubt."

We keep looking at the window.

After a deadly silence I say, "It's good to be on the first floor."

"Oh, no, yeah, so good. You're right there. So easy to find."

"And $6,000 a month? Considering? That's not..."

"Oh, no, yeah, it's not..."

"*That* much. Well, it's a lot, I mean, especially now, when we don't actually *have* six, you know, thousand dollars each and *every* month for five years and I don't have any patients yet...."

"*Yet*," Amy emphasizes.

More silence. Big silence. Deep silence.

"I'm just wondering," I say. "Thinking out loud. How do you think, you know, I will *get* patients?"

"You need to advertise," Amy says.

"Right," I say. "I can say I trained in Beverly Hills. That's a draw. That's a plus." I start to perk up. "I'll give my practice a sexy name. How's this?" I wave my hand in front of us, envisioning a large neon sign blinking over the front door of what will be my office. "The Beverly Hills Plastic Surgery Center of Rochester."

I speak the words slowly, reverentially, pausing powerfully after each syllable.

"What do you think?" I say.

"Well, it sounds, you know, a little, um, clunky," Amy says. "And a teeny bit...well, lame."

"What if I drop the *Rochester*?"

"Still."

"Yeah," I say. "Right."

Our eyes on the window, Amy reaches for my hand and entwines her fingers through mine.

"I love it here," I say again, trying to convince myself.

"I do too," she says, trying to convince me.

* * *

Good news, surprising news, *stellar* news travels fast.

Dr. Romeo Bouley and his plastic surgery dream team are going to be on national TV.

The hot new show on the *E!* Network, *Dr. 90210,* a reality series that shows actual plastic surgery procedures and follows doctors as if they're celebrities, has asked if they could film an episode with Dr. Bouley, Dr. George, and Dr. Bruce. Unfortunately, Dr. Bouley doesn't ask me to participate because, as Carla explains, he told the producers that by the time the show airs, I will be gone, self-banished to the backwaters of Michigan. I will no longer be part of their merry cast.

My heart sinks. Not only am I slightly starstruck (see my appearance on *Dick Clark's New Year's Rockin' Eve* followed by yet another TV appearance, also with Amy, this one on the *People's Choice Awards* as "seat fillers"), but I imagine that appearing on *Dr. 90210* will somehow benefit my new plastic surgery start-up. I'm not exactly sure how, but I know it will. Or at least I know it can't hurt.

I get the idea that *Dr. 90210* might want to film my good-bye party, which will be held in downtown LA at a Korean restaurant. I mention this to Carla, who mentions it to Dr. Bouley, who sees my good-bye party as a possible strong addition to the episode, a hook, adding drama and emotion, and tells me to write a letter to the producer. *Great,* I think, *the last one I wrote went out to thirty-three plastic surgeons in Michigan. Look how well that turned out.*

But I take Dr. Bouley's advice and write a letter, telling my story in melodramatic detail—Midwestern kid coming to LA, training in Beverly Hills, overcoming culture shock while honing my surgery skills, and then making the difficult decision to leave and head back to Michigan with no money, no patients, knee-buckling debt, hanging on to my dream of starting my own plastic surgery practice. The title of my sob story? *Young Korean American Doctor Makes Good Against All Odds.* Maybe. To be continued.

To my shock, the producer buys it.

He agrees to film my going-away party.

I rush to tell Dr. George, Dr. Bruce, and Carla the news. I know that Dr. George plays guitar and Carla sings, so I suggest that we play a song or two for the show. They love the idea. I rent a drum machine. We practice a couple of times to make sure that we won't suck and embarrass ourselves on national TV. We even give our impromptu band a name: SAG, short for Stephanie (Carla's middle name), Anthony, George.

The day of the going-away party the *Dr. 90210* crew first films me assisting a body lift with Dr. Bouley and Dr. George. While we clean up and change into our party clothes, the film crew interviews Amy. When I come into the room, they ask me questions for at least forty-five minutes.

We then head downtown for the party itself. The camera follows us through each moment of the party, the heartfelt toasts, the corny jokes, the good-bye and thank-you speeches, the two songs we play. At one point, Dr. Bouley looks deeply into the camera and says how fond he is of me and how much he'll miss me. I like to think he was totally sincere. Although he could've just been an incredibly convincing actor.

Finally, the film crew packs up and thanks us all. I calculate that *Dr. 90210* has shot at least two hours of footage, enough for two full shows. One of the crew, while winding a length of cable around his thick forearm, tells me that in his opinion this has been the best episode they've shot.

Stars sparkle in my eyes. My ego puffs out like a balloon. I see fan mail flooding my mailbox, paparazzi tracking me, shooting my picture as I disembark from The Ivy en route to my limo. I see myself jumping off the screen of that one episode and becoming a recurring character on the show. And then I see my own spinoff coming to America on the E! Network from my newly remodeled first-floor Beverly Hills Plastic Surgery Center office suite in Rochester, Michigan.

Wait for it.

I am *Dr. 48307*.

"When did they say they're going to air this?" I ask Dr. Bouley, clinking my beer bottle with his shot glass of Patron.

"They didn't," he says, slugging down his drink, swiping his lip with the back of his hand. "Maybe they never will."

I sip my beer.

My high spirits dissolve into the suds.

* * *

Sunday morning.

Moving day.

We pack everything we own into a U-Haul trailer that we hook up to our aging RAV4. Sad to say, we don't really have enough to fill the trailer halfway.

As we carry out the last of our boxes, mostly books, Dr. George, Dr. Bruce, and Carla arrive to see us off. They've brought a bottle of champagne. Our dog, Theodore, confused by the sudden emptying of our Westwood apartment, circles, barking nervously. He settles down and they talk of the future, mine and theirs. They've been discussing, mostly after hours with liquor-loosened lips, of going off on their own and starting their own practice. I'm not sure I believe them, but they're insistent that my leaving has served as their inspiration and motivation.

"The time is now," Dr. George says.

"To follow your dream," Dr. Bruce says, grim-faced, rubbing his hand along the side of the U-Haul.

"I'm gonna really miss you," Carla says, lowering her voice, eyeing Dr. George and Dr. Bruce. "You and I are the only normal ones."

"I heard that," Dr. Bruce says.

"It's sort of true," Dr. George says.

When we finish packing, Amy and I thank them for coming, and hug, lingering, murmuring inarticulate heartfelt good-byes and good lucks. They drive away and I choke back tears, aware suddenly of how much I'll miss those after-hours conversations at the Hamburger Hamlet and hanging out many nights and weekends. I didn't realize until this moment how close we'd become.

* * *

We drive next to Orange County, forty-five minutes away, to say good-bye to my parents.

We pull into the driveway of their small house and I see my parents waiting outside on the lawn. My mom holds a paper bag with sandwiches she's made. Like I'm ten years old. Still, I love it. My dad and I hug, saying little. Then he hugs and kisses Amy. As he wishes us luck, his lip quivers. He excuses himself and goes inside the house. He doesn't want us to see him cry.

My mom loses it then, tears gushing, her body shaking.

Naturally, as soon as she starts crying, Amy starts sobbing.

"Come on, you two," I say.

"I'm sorry," my mom says. "I can't help it."

"I can't either." Amy's crying ratchets up to match my mom's.

"Mom, we'll see you soon. You don't have to cry. This is a good thing."

"I'm not crying because I'm sad you're going," she says, struggling to speak through her sobs. "I'm crying because I'm sad that I don't have anything more to give you. Here."

She hands me an envelope.

"I wish I could give you more money than this, but with the stock market so bad and Daddy's retirement, this is all I have. I wanted to give you more. I always dreamed of giving you more, to help you get started."

"Mom, it's all right," I say. "Really. And you keep this." I push the slim envelope of money back into her hand.

"Don't insult me," she warns. "I want to give you what I can. So take it. Please."

I nod and accept the envelope from her, stuffing it into my shirt pocket. And then I hug her, breaking away before I too lose it.

"Make a good life," my mother says as we drive away. She stands on the lawn waving, refusing to go inside. The front door of the house opens and my dad comes out and stands next to her. As we drive away, I watch them in my rearview mirror, fading to small figures standing and waving on their front lawn.

We pull onto the freeway and hug the slow lane, the U-Hail trailer clattering behind us. I fiddle with the radio, settle on a station.

Billy Joel comes on and launches into "Say Goodbye to Hollywood."

Amy and I simultaneously start to sob. "Do you believe this?" I say, tears blinding me, swallowing sobs.

"No." Amy swabs her eyes, her cheeks, her nose. "Damn it."

"It's gonna be all right," I say through our crying and the rumble of the freeway.

"Yes," Amy says. "It's gonna be great."

"I have no patients, no prospects, and we have a ridiculous amount of debt," I sob.

"I know." Amy sobs.

I wail, Amy wails, Theodore howls from the back seat.

We drive east, into the unknown.

PART SEVEN

PRIVATE PRACTICE

16

Take My Card...*Please*

I'm a man on a mission.

I am going to take Detroit by storm.

I am going to *own* this town.

Doubt me?

Watch me!

After the strange and beautiful love I got from my peeps in the Beverly Hills plastic surgery community, but being brutally rejected by Detroit's old-line stodgy medical "establishment," I'm carrying a chip on my shoulder the size of a boulder. So now I'm going right to plan B. I will outwork, outwit, outfight, outthink, outlast, and out-everything anyone even resembling a doctor in town. I know that I'm starting in a deep, dark, cavernous hole, but that only fuels the fire in my belly and revs up the tiger in my tank. So what if I'm a quarter million dollars in debt? Who cares if I sent out thirty-three letters of introduction and nobody other than Dr. Paneer, who only wanted to rent me an operating room, and Dr. Wacko, who turned out to be a psycho, responded? Irrelevant.

And by the way, I don't want to merely insert myself into their Old Fart Doctor's Club. I don't want to be simply included. Oh, no, that wouldn't be victory enough. I want their business. I want to rip out their spleens with my sphygmomanometer, strangle them with my stethoscope, and destroy them with my tongue depressor. I want them to feel the fury of my wrath. I want them to suffer. I want them to come crying to me and beg for forgiveness. I want to napalm the old-line medical "establishment." I am Doctor Youn (almost rhymes with "Doom"), and you shall rue the day you rejected me!

OK, fine, so I've been reading a few too many comics and perhaps playing a few too many video games late into the night, but all that's out of my system now. Time to return those comics to their plastic wrappers, snap that controller in two, and implement my *plan*.

It's time!

Now all I have to do is actually come up with a plan.

I strategize, formulate and reformulate, and fine-tune. I get close. *Real* close. I think. Although actually, I'm not quite sure.

I, well, actually, Amy takes the first step, though, which really helps our cash flow. She gets a job.

Amy gets hired part-time as a pediatrician in a small practice, Tuesdays, Thursdays, and Fridays. When the partners realize what they have, they quickly lock her up full-time.

Meanwhile, I contact the contractor my landlord has hired to find out when he'll finish building out my office. He meets me there. We wander through the space, vacant and stark. It looks not only unfinished, but not actually started. He's already two weeks late. Eventually—hopefully soon—I will be performing reconstructive and cosmetic surgeries on, presumably, *people*, a lot of people, and the first impression they have of me means everything. Ergo, I need a nice office.

The contractor, an aloof, distracted guy, sports a bushy moustache that covers most of his face, no neck, and lumbering shoulders wide enough to haul a plow. He scratches his moustache—this requires both hands—and looks up at the sky, as if the answer to my question lies in the clouds, and says, "I'm behind."

"How, um, far behind?"

"Not my fault," he clarifies, lacquering up his moustache with a fistful of saliva. "It's the distributor and the lumberyard. Everything's on back order. Plus, electrical ran into permit issues. And plumbing? You don't even want to go there."

At that very moment, with the contractor covering us both with enough BS to fertilize everything east of the Mississippi, my usual easygoing, levelheaded nature dissolves right in front of my eyes. This man doesn't care if he craps on my parade. He's already gotten his down payment and won't give two pennies whether I have an office to see patients in. I need to stick up for myself so he doesn't bulldoze me. My heart races, my face flushes, and I gear up for a verbal fight.

"How *long*?" I peer into his pin-dot eyes stationed somewhere between his highway of hair and his Tigers ball cap.

The clouds above block the sun and we're engulfed in some dirty back-alley gray light, but the contractor is squinting like he's getting hit in the face with a laser beam.

"Need another six weeks," he mumbles, covering what I'm pretty sure is an ethnic slur.

"I can't wait any longer than that," I bark. "I have to be ready to move in by then. I should've been in by *now*." He wants to squint at me? Ha! I do my Korean version of the Clint Eastwood squint. "I'm serious. Dead serious."

I storm off cowboy style back to my rapidly rotting out RAV4 and dramatically swing open the door, get in, and slam the door so hard I'm afraid the tiny SUV will tip over.

But I'm on fire now. *En fuego*. And I attack.

I decide on a simple plan, simple as a shotgun blast, which I can sum up as: I have to get my name out there. Everywhere. People need to know that I *exist*. And I won't be ignored.

I apply to all the insurance companies. I will take any insurance, all insurance, every insurance, shady insurance sold on late-night TV, Medicare, Medicaid, any kind of aid, Kool-Aid—I'll drink it, whatever you got. I'll take it, guaranteed.

I apply to every hospital within an hour of my apartment. I'm willing to do the dirtiest of the dirty work. I offer to take emergency room calls. I offer to work any shift. I'm willing to go back to my old-time medical school, residency, no-sleep mode. I spent a year relaxing in the sunshine of Beverly Hills. I've slept enough. I'm not sleeping anymore. The giant has awoken. The kraken has been released.

I realize I need a temporary office for six weeks, giving my contractor the time he needs to finish my build-out. I call the local hospitals and medical centers and find a pain doctor who's willing to sublet his tiny office space—reception area and two small exam rooms—two half days a week, Monday and Wednesday mornings. Perfect. Amy's free. I check her availability and willingness and offer her unlimited bubble baths and massages. It works. In addition to being a brilliant pediatrician, she volunteers to become my office manager and receptionist. She'll book my appointments and greet and charm my patients. As soon as I have any. Ever the optimist, I purchase a portable credit card swiper and a plastic file cabinet on wheels. I create a logo and a small sign with my name and the name of my practice. I'm going with The Beverly Hills Plastic Surgery Center. I create a website and scrape together every penny I have and take out an ad in the *Yellow Pages.* The ad costs $1,000 a month. That's 100,000 pennies.

I also need furniture, medical supplies, malpractice insurance (I've learned the hard way that's a *must-have*), business insurance, decorations, and tons of other stuff to open an office. In addition, my malpractice carrier from Beverly Hills charges me $30,000 to cover the "tail" of the policy I had while there for a year. If I don't pay that amount they will no longer cover me for any lawsuits that may arise from my time in LA working with Dr. Bouley. After the "near-miss" lawsuit with Gina the Italian model, I decide there's no way I can go without it. Combined with the $6,000 I already paid the malpractice carrier, I come to the sober realization that all the money I made during my year in Beverly Hills will be spent on malpractice insurance.

I study my bank statement, sift through our bills, ogle the contractor's costs and overages, stare at Amy's salary, glower at my debt and balance sheets, and face this undeniable, hard-ass fact: I need a loan. I see no other way to finance my plastic surgery start-up. I sweat over my calculator and figure out the bare minimum I need to cover all my costs.

$130,000.

On top of the $250,000 I already owe.

I can't do it.

I can't add another $130,000 to my debt. It's insane and ridiculous and causes a vicious growling in my stomach like there's an alien in there champing at the bit to claw its way out.

I recalculate.

I cut this, trim that, eliminate this, postpone that.

Better.

$100,000.

I apply for a $100,000 loan at eleven banks.

Eleven turn me down.

All for the same reason.

I have nothing. No collateral. Zero history of any real income. Worse, I offer no actual promise of...anything. I'm eager, hardworking, skilled, well-educated, and the proud owner of a brand-new credit card swiper. Doesn't matter. No one will give me a loan.

I have one last bank to try and dupe into financing a man who has nothing, nowhere, and no one. I shine my shoes extra hard. I use extra deodorant and mouthwash. I say a brief but feverish prayer to God.

Miraculously, the officer at the last bank I contact, my last hope, my only hope, calls me and gives me a $100,000 line of credit.

To this day I have no idea why they come through when all the others turned me down.

At the time, I don't think about it.

I don't care.

I thank them profusely.

Yeah. Maybe I got the loan because I prayed to God. A lot.

Thanks, God.

* * *

I sit across from Amy at a breakfast place we like. I have decaf coffee, she has hot chocolate, we share a muffin. It's the starving-doctor breakfast special. In front of us sits a box of five hundred business cards I've just picked up from the printer. Amy looks at one, turns it over, tests the paper stock, smiles, nods, hands it back to me.

"I like it. Simple, classy, easy to read."

"The corners are sharp and flexible too, so if you don't have a toothpick..." She laughs, a little. I sigh. "OK. *Well...*"

She takes my hands and gives me her classic Amy you-can-do-this look. "Don't be discouraged. You're just getting started."

"I know. That wasn't a sigh of discouragement. That was my *I'm gearing up to kick some serious butt, gonna wrassle me up about a million patients who need plastic surgery, dawg* look."

"Now *that's* what I'm talking about."

"So, to recap: Got my ad running, taking call at all the local emergency departments, and talking up my practice to anyone who will listen. But bottom line, I gotta take my message to the people. I gotta hit the mean streets of Rochester and the rest of

Detroit hard. Educate the public. My goal? I vow to give out at least one card a day."

"Ambitious. Go for it."

Our waitress floats over and refills my coffee cup. She's a tired-looking woman in her sixties. Her skin sags. Her eyes droop. Flab jiggles around her neck. She could definitely benefit from a little plastic surgery pick-me-up. I look at Amy. She looks back, amused, and rests her chin on a steeple of her folded hands. She offers no information, confirmation, or encouragement. The gauntlet has been thrown down. I'm on my own here. I catch the waitress's nametag. Irene.

"How you doing today, Irene?" I say.

She raises a thick eyebrow. "Fine. For a Monday."

"I'd like to introduce myself. I'm Doctor Tony Youn. I'm kind of new in town. I do plastic surgery. Here's my card. I was wondering if you, or anyone you know, a friend, family member, might consider me to be their doctor...."

Irene's face rolls into a terrifying frown, the kind of glower that precedes a hard left hook to the chin. "You think I need plastic surgery? You think I'm ugly? Is that what you think?"

"Oh, no, no, no. I didn't mean it that way. I only meant..."

"I like the way I look."

"Oh, no, no, no, yes, you look *fine*. More than fine. You look very...pretty. And presentable. And clean. And excellent. You look excellent. Awesome even. You personally wouldn't need any plastic surgery that I can see, of course, but you never know...."

"Excuse me!" Irene storms off and blows through the swinging double doors into the kitchen. I hear a shrill wail, a cross between a caw and a sob.

I absentmindedly rub the side of the box of cards. "She didn't take the card, so I won't count her."

"Yeah, no, I wouldn't," Amy says. "And just a thought. You may want to tweak your pitch."

* * *

I don't let Irene the waitress discourage me. Later that day I offer cards to my waitress at the lunch place and then to the woman working the counter at the donut shop and to the two young baristas with facial piercings at Starbucks. They all reject my cards. Some more politely than others. Over the next week, I discover that, in general, waitresses seem offended when I ask if they're interested in taking a plastic surgeon's business card. I might as well be leading with the line "Can I interest you in a breath mint?"

Amy's right. I have to work on my pitch.

I decide to expand my circle of potential patients. I give my card out to people at the pharmacy, the office supply store, the bookstore, the grocery store. I get suspicious frowns, sarcastic grins, one or two out-and-out guffaws. A couple of people who look like they want to punch my lights out. I decide to focus my card giveaways on more likely candidates. I pass my card out at the gym. The next day I go to a different gym and the day after that I go to the Y and pass out cards to the people working out and working the front desk. I give my card out at the hair salon. Then three weeks later, when I get my hair cut again, I go to a different salon and pass my card out there. Two weeks after that I get another haircut, even though I don't need one, and go to yet another salon so I can pass my card out to a whole new group of hair people.

At night I sit at my crappy computer on our wobbly card table we bought for five dollars at a garage sale and churn out letters to every local chapter of every organization I can think of within a fifty-mile radius. The Rotary Club, the Lions Club, the Elks Club, the Moose Club, the Shriners, the orchestra guild, the library association, the historical society, the Medieval Reenactment Club, knitting circles, swingers clubs, churches, synagogues, young Democrats and Republicans, old Democrats and Republicans—and offer them a free talk on the latest in plastic surgery. I offer to donate any honorariums to charity. I get an immediate response from the Rotarians. I set up a time—my calendar is wide open, but I play it cool and tell them I have to move some stuff around—and drive over to a community center where the Rotary Club holds its monthly meetings.

As I walk into the lobby, the receptionist, Sonya, greets me with a suspicious-looking mole on her cheek. I'm at the point where I can hear the mole talking to me. *Tony, dude, you gotta get me out of here. Tell her you can get rid of me. Her health insurance will cover it.* I'm tempted to hand her my card, but I restrain myself. I'll talk with her later, after I wow the audience with my talk.

"So nice of you to come, Doctor Youn," she says. "We've gotten a nice turnout. I'd say we have forty people in there."

"That's great. More than I would've thought," I say, trying to blink away the images of a full waiting room dancing in front of my eyes.

"Oh, we have a very active membership," Sonya says.

"Terrific." I tighten my tie, shoot my cuffs through the jacket of my only suit, and enter the auditorium convinced this is the moment when my practice, and my life, finally take off.

As Sonya promised, forty people eagerly await my talk....

Thirty-six men.

Four women.

Average age: eighty-three.

Not exactly my target demographic.

I talk to them for my allotted time, forty-five minutes, about new techniques in the field of plastic surgery. I'm enthusiastic, animated, and, most important, loud. I think the talk goes over really well because I hear a minimum of snoring and no one passes away. After a brief Q and A, I circulate among the crowd and pass out forty-three cards.

By the end of the week, I learn that the Rotarians loved my talk so much that Sonya has recommended me to the Lions Club, whose president calls to schedule a talk there. I accept. I talk to the Lions Club. Average age of the Lions: eighty-three. And to the Elks Club and the Shriners and the orchestra guild. Average age of the Elks, Shriners, and orchestrans: eighty-three. In all, I talk to a dozen clubs and organizations. Average age? You guessed it. Eighty-three. I am the keynote speaker in heaven's waiting room. I receive warm applause and phone numbers pressed into my hand from a dozen people who want me to call their daughters. And one phone number from a woman who wants me to call her son. I'm a business-card-distributing fool. In fact, I distribute so many business cards that I have to go back to the printer and order another five hundred. The result of these talks? I receive exactly no calls for consultations or appointments.

None. Zero. Nada. *Niente*. Zilch. Not a single one.

I go back to the folding table and write letters to every family doctor and internist I can find within thirty miles. I include a business card with the letter.

I receive exactly the same number of responses.

Zero point zero.

I decide that letters are too impersonal, too cold. I need to press the flesh.

I show up at the first family doctor's office on my list with bagels, a tub of cream cheese, and two gallons of orange juice. I am Mr. Congeniality as I introduce myself to the receptionist and ask if I might speak to the doctor for five minutes, just to say hi.

"Oh, so nice of you to stop by. And bagels. Yum. Just put them and the orange juice in that room over there and have a seat. I'm sure the doctor will stop by between patients. *So* nice of you."

I thank her, place my forty dollars' worth of bagels, cream cheese, and orange juice in the back room, take a seat, and wait. And wait. After an hour of being ignored, I think, *What the hell am I doing? I'm a doctor, not some salesman. I'm a freaking doctor.*

The words screaming in my head, I'm tempted to grab what's left of my bagels, cream cheese, and orange juice offering and leave.

The cooler, calmer voice in my head prevails. Instead, I just leave.

I wake up the next morning, buy another forty dollars' worth of orange juice and bagels, and hit another family doctor's office.

Same result.

This is ridiculous, I think after an hour, my leg bobbing up and down, making the polished wood floor simultaneously squeak and vibrate. I feel like a fool. Not to mention that I'm out eighty dollars and I never got a bite of a bagel or a sip of juice. I leave and vow never to do this again.

I stick to my vow. Almost. I drag my sorry butt to three more doctors' offices armed with my alms of bagels and orange juice before I throw in the towel.

Two hundred dollars.

Flushed.

Down the toilet.

* * *

I silk screen a T-shirt with my name, address, phone number, and website on it. I create what I think is a cool design and logo and make up a dozen T-shirts in several color combinations. I wear the T-shirt everywhere. I wear it to work out, to run, to walk the dog, to restaurants, to the grocery store, even to a T-shirt store. People like the T-shirt. They comment on it. They tell me they like the design, the logo, the color combinations, the website.

Nobody calls for an appointment.

Nobody.

* * *

God bless the *Yellow Pages.*

A woman sees my ad and calls me. She tells me that her name is Blossom and she's calling from Detroit. All calls on my office number automatically go to my cell phone. I'm driving back from my fourth haircut that day (or so it seems), where I've handed out business cards at yet another salon.

"I saw your ad," Blossom says.

"Hold on a moment, please," I say, and pull over to the side of the road. I try not to hyperventilate as I hold the phone in two hands and attempt to tamp down the quivering excitement that's shooting through the nerves in my fingers. "Yes, this is Doctor Youn."

"You do implants?"

"Yes, uh-huh, absolutely."

"I want a butt implant."

"A—what now?"

"Butt implant. I want a big-ass booty."

I pause. "I don't really...I've never...Well, what I *can* do is liposuction."

"Liposuction? I don't want *liposuction*. I don't want to take nothing out. I want a big-ass booty. Do you or do you not do booty implants?"

I pause again and negotiate with myself. I've never done a butt implant. But what the heck? Dead-broke panic can be the mother of invention. I can stick an implant in a butt. Can't I?

"I'll tell you what. Why don't you come in for a consultation and we'll talk about it? We'll figure out what you need, what's best for you, and we'll go from there. How does that sound?"

"That sounds good. OK. I'll make an appointment."

"Great! Terrific. Wonderful. Let me just get my book...." I reach into my bag, my fingers still shaking with excitement, and accidentally fling my address book into the back seat. I curse under my breath, stretch over the passenger seat, and retrieve my calendar. "OK, then, I have availabilities..." Basically, every second for the rest of my life. "Either next Monday morning or next Wednesday morning. How about Monday at nine?"

"Monday at nine. That'll work."

"Excellent." I give Blossom my address, thank her for calling, hang up the phone, pump my fist, and scream,

"Score!"

My voice echoes off the tin walls of my RAV4, blasting through every ounce of my being.

Blossom.

My first patient.

I thank God for my first break.

* * *

Blossom never shows.

I wait one hour. I call her, get her voice mail. I leave a message, repeat my address. I wait another hour. I have to go. The doctor whose office I'm subletting has an appointment. I pack up my plastic file cabinet on rollers, slip my portable credit card swiper into my bag, leave the office, and take down my portable sign, my shoulder sagging, my heart dragging, like a plastic surgeon version of the perpetually depressed donkey Eeyore from *Winnie the Pooh*.

Blossom.

I never hear from her again.

* * *

I go over our finances.

Sinking fast.

I am the *Titanic* of unemployed plastic surgeons.

I've nearly exhausted our teeny tiny savings and I'm burning through the $100,000 loan I took out like it's kindling. I need to bring in some money, anything, to keep us afloat. I sidle up to the computer on the card table that acts as my desk and office and again start writing letters, this time to urgent care centers. I offer to diagnose sore throats and coughs, put in and remove stitches, lance ass boils, drain colostomy bags, anytime, day, night, weekends, Christmas Eve, Yom Kippur, whenever or wherever. I expand my geographical range to anything within a hundred miles.

I receive no responses.

Zero point zero.

I look over the letter. Is it inarticulate? Is it offensive?

Maybe I'm overqualified. A real plastic surgeon applying to work in urgent care.

* * *

Finally, one evening the phone rings.

It's a doc I know who works in a clinic in Grand Rapids, a two-and-a-half-hour drive away. He has something for me. I can work at his clinic, one night a week, for three hours a night. He'll pay me $150. I do some quick, painful math. It will cost me at least twenty bucks for gas, probably more, plus I will have to get a hotel room. Even if he pays me under the table, I won't bring in more than fifty dollars for the night. *Ughh,* I think, balancing risk and reward. *Is it worth the drive? Absolutely not.*

"I'll take it," I say.

Fifty dollars may not be a ton of money, but it's better than selling my own plasma and reproductive fluids.

The following week, two other clinics call. They have nothing right now, but in three months they anticipate personnel change-over and they may have something for me. They promise to call.

I thank them, thrilled at the promise, but knowing that a promise won't pay my bills.

* * *

It must be the name.

The Beverly Hills Plastic Surgery Center.

It's putting people off. It sounds too...pretentious.

And it may be confusing people. It sounds too...out of state. Don't want GPS sending patients to California.

I need to change it to something closer to home.

Rochester Plastic Surgery Center.

Nah. Too bland. I have to go for something catchier. Sexier. Got it.

A Cut Above.

Uggh. Sounds like a place to get a cheap haircut.

Doctor Youn's Perfect Tens.

Yuck. Too strip clubby. Makes me want to take a shower and wash off all the glitter.

Ah. Here we go. It's mysterious, cool, inviting.

Y.P.S.

Get it?

Youn Plastic Surgery.

Clever, no?

Not really.

Pondering while I pump gas, leaning against the passenger door of my increasingly decrepit RAV4, the little SUV creaks, groans, and shakes even as I fuel it up. I sigh and run my fingers through my hair. Not much there. The last thing I need is a haircut, but I have an appointment scheduled in an hour at yet another hair salon so I can hand out more business cards to unsuspecting stylists and manicurists and hair washers who couldn't care less about getting plastic surgery or referring me to any of their clients. I consider canceling. I'm not getting anywhere passing out business cards to random people. And if I decide to change the name of my practice, the business cards will be worthless anyway. Great. Another hundred bucks to print new cards. Perfect. Money's leaking through my hands like really expensive bottled water.

I glance across the pump at the guy on the other side. He's a trucker wearing a faded lumberjack shirt with a denim vest over that. He's enormous, six-four or six-five, weighing two fifty at least, with two hundred of it belly. He wears a full red Viking beard and what looks like a permanent scowl. He grunts as he tops off the gas tank of his semi and returns the nozzle to its perch in the pump. We make eye contact. I smile and nod. He grunts and sniffs.

And then I see it.

The mole from hell.

Huge. A raised rough black growth the size of a half-dollar on his forehead.

I blink to be sure I'm not hallucinating from the gas fumes.

No. It's there. It's real. And definitely cancerous.

The trucker waddles toward the driver's side of his semi.

I click off pumping my gas, return my nozzle to its pump, and run toward the trucker, heading him off. "Excuse me, sir."

He stops and glares at me. "What?"

"Well, that mole."

I wait a moment for him to respond. He looks at me like he'd enjoy rearranging my face.

"Look, I'm a plastic surgeon," I say a little breathlessly. "I just wanted you to know that if you're interested I could take that off for you. If you have insurance, that would be great. But even if you don't..."

"What the hell are you talking about?"

"The mole, sir. Your *mole.*" I point my thumb at it as if I'm hitchhiking. "You really have to deal with it. There's a good chance it could be cancerous." I fumble in my shirt pocket. "Here's my card. Call me. I'm not trying to alarm you, but it could be serious."

He squints at my card. "Beverly Hills Plastic Surgery?"

"Yeah, I know. I'm gonna change the name...."

"I don't have time for this crap!" The Viking trucker slams the card back into my hand.

This time I'm upset that someone hasn't taken my card.

This time it's different.

This time I could actually be saving a man's face. Or his life.

I press him. "Listen, sir, please. You really need to have that looked at."

He waves at me dismissively, lumbers back into the cab of his semi, and revs his engine. I step back as he and his mole roar out of the gas station without looking back at me.

Every now and then I think about him and pray that he's OK.

* * *

Time flies by. August comes through hot and sticky, gives way to an even hotter and stickier early September. As the heat outside flattens me and the end of summer approaches, a nasty cocktail of gloom and depression consumes me.

I spend too many days sitting at the card table at our tiny apartment, plowing through paperwork, planning talks, writing letters, and strategizing about ways to get my practice going. But mostly I sit impotent, waiting for the phone to ring, be it from a potential patient or from a clinic offering me anything—the graveyard shift, *anything*.

Nothing.

The phone gathers dust. The silence chokes me. The highlight of my day becomes the fifteen minutes I take Theodore for a walk. My trusty, slightly overweight shih tzu has become my best buddy, my companion, my confidant, my business partner in a business where there's no business. On sunny days we sit on the tiny apartment patio together for hours, him sleeping on and off, and me in a folding chair hammering away at my laptop. He listens, or seems to, as I lament and worry, his large brown eyes not understanding a thing I say but offering his unwavering loyalty and support.

The build-out of my office has also hit a snag. The owner of the building informs me that the contractor needs more time, at least two more weeks. Most of the time I don't have the strength or energy to call the contractor and make a pest of myself. I know he and his buddies are laughing at me, thinking I'm just a clueless

Asian doctor whom he can easily manipulate and swindle. The one time I do call, as soon as I identify myself, the contractor makes a loud, fake, scratchy noise with his throat, tells me he's driven into a bad cell area, he's losing me, and hangs up. Dejected, I don't call back. I fear that his assessment of me is right.

And then, one day, a miracle.

I get a call from Hollywood.

17

Dr. 90210

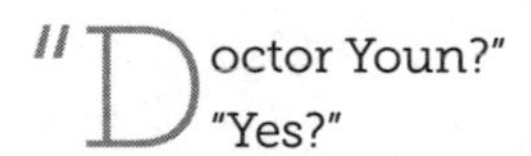

"Doctor Youn?"

"Yes?"

"This is Suzy. I'm calling from the *E!* Network. I'm an assistant producer on *Dr. 90210*?"

"Oh, hi, I'd almost forgotten about that show."

"Well, I wanted to tell you that the episode you filmed is going to air Sunday."

Panic.

That's what I feel.

Not relief, not excitement, not joy, not hope...

Panic.

"You mean *this* Sunday? As in five days from now?"

"Yes."

"Wow, OK, that's great, very exciting, and so very...*soon.*"

"That's why I'm calling. We've already aired one episode and the response has been extremely positive. Ratings are through the roof. And between us, I just screened your episode. You're awesome. You steal the whole half hour."

"I do? I steal it? Seriously?"

"Oh, totally. You're amazing. So, yeah, I wanted to give you a heads up so you can alert your people."

"My...people?"

I look over at Theodore. He sniffs his butt.

I then count my people.

Amy and Theodore.

I have very few people.

"Yeah, you know," Suzy says, "your agent, your manager, your publicist, or whoever you use for this sort of thing?"

"Ah, yes, of course. I'll call my publicist, and my...manager, yes, my manager—and my other...*people*—right now. Thank you."

I hang up. Theodore yawns. Sniffs his butt again.

"I know," I say to him. "You're the only one around here who actually has people."

* * *

I call Amy, who screams over the phone, probably scaring the crap out of all the kids in the waiting room. I remember for the billionth time why I married her.

"We have to get the word out," she says. "Maybe we should hire a publicist. What am I saying? That would cost money. Forget that."

"We don't need no stinking publicist," I say. "I'm on it."

I hang up, fire up the computer, and google "How to write a press release."

I find a step-by-step guide online and write my first ever press release announcing that I, Dr. Anthony Youn, from Rochester's very own Beverly Hills Plastic Surgery Center—such a great name—will be appearing on the hot new reality show *Dr. 90210.* After I'm sure I've created the perfect press release, I do something I never do—I sleep on it. In the morning, I read the press release over, and I'm shocked at how bad it is. I throw out half of it, rewrite it, punch it up. Then, in a completely unprecedented move, I sleep on it again. The third day I reread it. It doesn't seem like the big piece of crap I thought it was, so I make a few minor changes and fax it to every TV and radio station in the metro Detroit area. I send it everywhere.

Within an hour, the producer of a local radio show called *Motor City Middays* phones me. He invites me to appear on the show Monday morning at ten o'clock, a hot time because the show follows Howard Stern.

For the first time since we moved to Michigan, I feel a shift. At the end of the black hole tunnel I've been in, I see a tiny flickering light. My depression lifts. My energy level shoots sky high. I feel that I am on my way. Doctor Youn's back in the saddle, baby! And ready to rock 'n' roll.

Amy and I celebrate by going out to dinner.

"I don't want to overstate it," I say, "but this is big."

"Huge. National TV. Ridiculous."

"It's my debut."

"Let's have a viewing party," she says. "We'll have, like, a Hollywood premiere."

"Awesome," I say. "We'll invite all our friends."

"Absolutely," she says. Then she pauses and thinks. "One problem. We don't have any friends."

Sunday night at ten o'clock, all my people are gathered. Amy and Theodore cuddle with me on our couch, Amy and I sipping cheap champagne, Theodore gnawing on a shiny new chew toy we bought him for the occasion. We tune our bulbous stone-age seventeen-inch TV onto the E! Network. The theme music swells. The opening credits appear. Amy and I applaud. Theodore barks. My excitement builds. The show starts. For the first ten minutes, we see no sign of me.

And then, there I am, unrecognizable in green scrubs, my name superimposed on the bottom of the screen for approximately 1.3 seconds over the legs of the operating table.

"The producer person said I stole the show," I mumble miserably.

"Be patient," Amy says. "I'm sure you're the grand finale."

The show's minutes and commercials tick by.

I no longer appear to be in the show at all and I'm all out of patience. My heart racing, my disappointment so palatable even Theodore nervously puts aside his chew toy and pants sympathetically, I spring off the couch and pace.

Finally, with about three minutes left in the half-hour program, the setting shifts to the Korean restaurant we all went to for my going-away party.

And there I am, smiling on camera, speaking directly to Dr. Romeo Bouley.

"Thank you for teaching me how to be a Beverly Hills plastic surgeon," I say, my sincerity surprising even to me.

Dr. Bouley, twirling a nearly empty wineglass by its stem, faces all of us at home and says, "You know, I made him an offer he couldn't refuse, and he refused it. He's going back to Rochester, Michigan."

That's it.

That's my entire national television appearance.

Less than thirty seconds of screen time.

The closing credits crawl, music goes quiet, the show fades to black. As do my hopes. Amy clears her throat, Theodore hops onto the floor and curls into a fetal position by his water bowl. I'm tempted to do the same. Instead, I throw myself back onto the couch, sigh what feels like a death rattle, and stare at the ceiling.

"I liked what I saw," Amy, ever my cheerleader, says with what seems like genuine enthusiasm.

"Oh, yeah, I was splendid," I say. "All thirty seconds of me. Good thing we didn't have any friends to invite over."

I rest my champagne flute on the floor beside me where a coffee table should be. Before viewing the show, I had visions of sometime in the future being able to afford a coffee table. I have visions of the rest of my life spent here, at the rickety card table, trying to devise a plan C or a plan D, counting the minutes until it's time for Theodore's walk.

"Not what I expected," I say.

"What did you expect?"

"A game changer."

* * *

Eight o'clock the next morning. Monday. My cell phone rings, the ringtone telling me it's my office number. Amy, selecting Monday as her day off from work, snatches the phone and answers in her official receptionist's voice: "Doctor Youn's office." She raises an eyebrow in shocked surprise, as she scribbles what appears to be an appointment into my calendar. She hangs up, starts to say something, and is interrupted when the phone rings again. By the time I leave for my appearance on *Motor City Middays*, she's scheduled five new consultations.

I keep waiting to wake up at the rickety card table, looking down at Theodore waiting for me to take him for his afternoon constitutional.

I don't wake up. This is really happening. I have five new patients.

Five new patients!

I don't come on the radio show until the final hour, but I'm on for the entire time and the hosts shamelessly plug me and my practice. When I get home after the show, I ask Amy what she thought of my interview. "I didn't really hear it," she says. "I was too busy answering the phone and making appointments. We've got fifteen new consultations. One woman said, 'I only want Doctor Youn to do my surgery.' I told her I'd have to make sure you were available."

We whoop. We holler. We do our victory dance in our apartment.

Fifteen new freaking consultations!

The phone calls don't stop that day. The next day I book a dozen more consultations, answering one call at Walmart as I'm walking down an aisle behind a frazzled mother and her two kids who are pushing each other.

"Hello? Doctor Youn's office. May I help you?" I say cheerily, trying to disguise my voice.

A female voice answers back. "Yes, I'd like to make an..."

"Stop touching me!" the boy yells to his sister, who then drops a jar of tomato sauce on the floor.

Crash! Both children begin screaming.

I fumble with my cell phone, trying to cover the microphone.

"Damn kids! I'll give you something to cry about!" the mother screams.

"Hello?" the patient says. "Am I still on with Doctor Youn's office? I'm trying to schedule an appointment...."

"Oh, no, yes, this is Doctor Youn's office," I say, scrambling away from the bedlam, trying in vain to make this sound like the hottest new plastic surgery office in Metro Detroit.

"Clean up in aisle six!" a clerk announces overhead.

"Excuse me? What's going on?"

"I'm sorry, but we must've gotten our lines crossed or...something. I'd be happy to make you an appointment to see Doctor Youn," I say, stepping over a puddle of marinara sauce.

* * *

Consultations! Pouring in! Whaaaaaaat?!

I see my very first real patient—a guy with pronounced gynecomastia, aka man boobs—scheduled for a Monday morning at nine fifteen.

Amy—my nurse/office manager/receptionist—and I arrive at nine. I carry my plastic file folder and Amy holds our credit card swiper (the one I was beginning to think I'd never get to actually use) as I hang my temporary sign on the door. I try the door. Locked. In what I now call a moment of shortsightedness, but which in actuality is just raw naked stupidity, I never thought to ask the pain doctor to give me my own key. So, as usual, I have to wait for the office receptionist to arrive. She is, as usual, late. I check my watch. Nine fifteen.

"She's always late," I mutter.

"She'll be here," Amy says.

"Yeah, I know. I just want her to arrive before my first real patient ever—*Jerry!*"

A large man, his pendulous chesticles swishing and swaying beneath the African tunic he's wearing, walks toward us. "Good morning, Doctor Youn."

"How you doing?" I smile like an idiot, trying not to look as stupid as I feel.

"I'm OK. A little, you know, nervous."

Me too, I don't say.

"I can understand that, but I promise, you have nothing to worry about."

"Oh, you're in really good hands," Amy says. "Literally."

Nobody makes a move toward the door. We stand there, idiotically, the three of us, silently waiting.

"Why are we standing here?" Jerry finally asks. "Why aren't we, you know, going inside?"

"We," I try not to sound too pissed, "don't have a key."

"Oh," Jerry says, nodding, drying his sweaty palms on his tunic. He frowns, looks at my plastic file folder and the portable credit card swiper Amy cradles in her arms. "Isn't this your office?"

"It is!" I say too loudly, then quickly lower my voice into confident doctor mode. "Monday and Wednesday mornings. It's a sublet. I'm waiting for the contractor to finish building out my regular office. He's a tad behind schedule."

"Well, I don't care," Jerry says, slapping his enormous man boobs. "Just get rid of these tatas. And if possible, I'd prefer that you not do the surgery with a rusty steak knife in the parking lot."

"No promises," I say, all of us laughing, and then, finally, thankfully, the receptionist pulls up in her car.

I'm grateful that Jerry has a sense of humor and doesn't walk out on me.

Thanks, Jerry.

* * *

I quickly outgrow the sublet.

I simply have too many patients.

It's a day I never thought I'd see.

I'm booked beyond my Monday and Wednesday morning schedule.

I also have an image to protect.

I can't afford word to get out that I'm anything less than worthy of my flashy brand: the Beverly Hills Plastic Surgery Center. After all, I've starred (well, appeared) on national TV. OK, it was only for thirty whole seconds. But still, I don't want people to think that I'm some sketchy, fly-by-night doc-in-a-box with a temporary office and erratic hours. I have to make some changes.

I need my *office*.

I call the contractor. He's months behind. I tell him I can't wait anymore. I've got patients backed up. I'm losing time. I'm losing money.

"I hear you, man," he says like he really means it. All evidence to the contrary. "It's gotta be tough."

"It *is* tough. I have to move into my office. When are you going to be done?"

"End of September. That's a promise."

OK, I think. That's only three weeks away. "Seriously? You promise?"

"That's more than a promise. A guarantee."

End of September arrives. My office remains an empty shell. When I walk through my twelve hundred square feet of nothingness, it's obvious that it's sat untouched for months. I'm steamed. I call the contractor. "You said end of September. What's going on?"

He blows out a sympathetic sigh. "Circumstances out of my control. Major problems at the factory. Union stuff. And then there was that industrial accident? The guy who lost both feet? I'm sure you read about that, was in all the papers..."

"Listen, I have to get into my office. I can't wait anymore."

"Oh, no, yeah, I get that. Totally. And I'm on it. I'm gonna be in there all weekend. Gonna slam it. And, Doc, the best news? It's gonna be amazing. A showplace. Worth the wait."

"So, you're gonna be in there all weekend?"

"Yes, sir. Twenty-four seven. Until we finish."

"OK, then that'll be fine."

I show up Saturday.

Nobody's there.

I wait an hour.

Nobody shows.

I leave, come back two hours later.

Nobody. I stare at the blank walls. I call the contractor on his cell.

"Hey, it's Doctor Youn..."

"Wait, what? I'm in a bad area...."

He hangs up.

I call him back.

His phone goes straight to voice mail.

I wait a half hour and call back.

No answer.

I *67 him so he can't see who's calling. He picks up. "Yo, Dude, you got the beer?"

"No, I don't. It's Doctor Youn. What is going on with my office?"

"Oh, hey, Doctor Youn. My cell's been acting crazy. Yeah, listen. The guys got hung up. There's like a twenty-five-car pileup on I-75. They'll be there. Gonna bust all weekend, brother. Gonna *crush* it."

I wait two more hours and go back to the office.

Nobody. Nothing.

I don't have the heart or the strength to call the contractor again. I go home, deflated. Years of crushing medical school. Sleepless years of soul-sucking residency. Months of giving dozens of talks without a single call back. Yet nothing prepared me for the horrors of the contractor. He is gutting me. I'd find another contractor, but I've already paid the first a hefty sum and have no money to hire someone else.

I return to the office Sunday.

Empty.

I vacillate between blinding rage and utter impotence.

I call the contractor Monday.

"I'm sorry, man," he says. "The guys flaked on me. Blindsided me. They promised. You should never hire family or guys who hang out at Home Depot, right? Ha, ha, *ha*! I'm kidding. Anyway. Listen, you have my word. We're gonna work all week. And you have to know this. Your office is my number one priority. Numero uno."

"I'm gonna hold you to that."

"Oh. Yes, sir. You have my word."

Nobody shows up during the week.

Nobody shows up the following weekend.

I call the contractor every day, twice a day. I call him during work hours and in the evening. Most of my calls go to voice mail.

When we do talk, he promises to complete my remodel within the next week.

Nobody ever shows up. And it's always going to get done *next* week.

I will give him this. His excuses become more inventive, more elaborate, more colorful.

His crew started the work on the wrong building, his dog ate all the contracts, and now he claims to be recovering from a sudden case of mad cow disease.

Finally, beyond the end of my tether, I call the owner of the building. I am done with this.

"Hey, Doctor Youn, how are you doing?"

"Not great. I'm pulling out of my lease. You promised to have my office completed months ago. The contractor hasn't even started. I'm out."

"You can't do that."

"I can and I will."

"All right, look, calm down. I really want you in that building. Let me get back to you."

"You don't have to get back to me. If my office isn't finished in one week, I'm pulling out and you'll get a call from my lawyer."

This last part slips out, but I don't mind. *Nice touch*, I think, especially since I don't have a lawyer. I don't even know a lawyer.

"OK, all right, don't panic. I will get it done."

To my shock, he does.

A week after I call, I open the door to my formerly vacant cold space and enter an actual waiting room of an actual—office. Totally completed.

Well...

As I recover from the elation of actually having an office, I realize it's a shoddy mess.

They've put up the wrong wallpaper.

They've built mismatched cabinets that don't quite fit.

They've chosen wood framing and door jambs in dark cherry and built cabinets of light maple. They more than clash. They trade body blows. They're eyesores that send you off into the light, blinking.

The owner calls me. He gushes over the phone. "Told you I'd get it done. Gorgeous, isn't it?"

"No," I say.

"No?"

I list the litany of mistakes the contractor has made. But despite my best intentions, my voice trails off weakly. I have, in fact, lost the will to fight. Instead, I focus on the larger picture: patients who need to be seen in my office, people who have appointments, individuals to whom I've made promises. I don't love what the dirtbag contractor's built, but I'll live with it. More than that, even though it largely sucks, it's mine.

I go to Furniture Express and buy the furniture I need, all at clearance center prices. I have the fashion sense of an aging boxer with detached retinas, so I purchase everything in blue. That way I know all the couches, chairs, and exam tables will at least match. I choose blue because that's the color I've used in my logo. I also read online that psychologists consider blue to be the most soothing color. Plus, it's a "boy color," and I'm a boy. I spend dozens of hours putting the cheap furniture together myself, even staining the wood of my exam tables. And then, finally, I receive an unexpected gift.

My last day at the sublet, I perform a consultation on a lovely woman who's seeing me for fat injections to treat complications from a previous surgery. She seems a little ill at ease.

"Are you OK?" I ask her.

"I'm fine. I was just wondering—well, you're new here and all—are you by any chance hiring? I'm looking for an office position."

"Wow. Timing," I say. "My wife just quit."

"Oh, I'm sorry...."

"No, no, it's fine. It was planned. She's going to work full time. But, yes, sure, you're hired."

OK, so I'm not exactly Terry Gross when it comes to interviewing.

"Really? Great!"

"Can you start tomorrow?"

"Don't you want to see my résumé or check my references or..."

"Of course, yeah, at some point...."

"You want to look at my résumé *after* you hire me?"

"Well, you're trustworthy, aren't you? I'm sure you're good at your job, right?" I realize as I'm saying this that I am possibly the *worst* hirer in the history of hiring.

"Yes, of course, absolutely." She looks a little worried. "Well, about the surgery..."

"You'll be fine. And if not, you'll be five feet away from a follow-up with me."

At last, with mismatched cabinets, a calming blue color scheme, and one employee whom I hired on the spot, with no résumé, no background check, during the middle of a consultation, I open my doors full time.

18

Driving in Neutral

We celebrate at Lipuma's, the local Coney Island hot dog restaurant. As we dig into our dogs, Amy and I finalize what we refer to as our five-year plan.

We'll live on her income and use the money that comes in from my (hopefully) burgeoning new practice to chip away at and ultimately exterminate our crippling debt—the $250,000 we've accrued from college and medical school loans and the $100,000 line of credit I took from the one bank that dared believe I wasn't a joke or a deadbeat or both. We vow to live with frugal joy, purchasing just the bare necessities, and spending nothing (or next to it) on ourselves until we're out of hock. We toast to the future and our promise to squirrel away as much money as possible. We seal it with a clink of our water cups and a kiss.

Wiping my lip with my napkin, I decide this is absolutely the worst time to talk about buying a new car. I don't consider myself particularly materialistic. I like owning nice things as much as the next person, but I don't crave a custom-made Lamborghini or the latest and the greatest bejeweled iPhone. And I don't judge people by the amount or quality of stuff they own. I'm not that shallow.

But here's the thing.

I drive a crappy car.

An old crappy car.

God bless the RAV4. She was a good old soldier, but at this point, she's not even a nice old crappy car. She's a rusted-out, groaning, moaning piece of junk mini SUV that even minivans laugh at. She's got tires balder than Steve Harvey. I won't bring up buying new tires because according to our business plan, we can't afford to, even though winter is not just coming, it has arrived.

Let's be honest.

I do not drive a "doctor's car."

And I am, in fact, a doctor. A doctor who's smart enough not to initiate that conversation because I know it will quickly dissolve into an analysis of my image and my desire to "look the part." I don't want to go there. I'll say this, though, just between us. I do believe I have an image to protect. I think that if you look successful, people assume you *are* successful. And when it comes to selecting a doctor to perform their plastic and reconstructive surgery, people will go with who appears to be the most successful. We are, after all, talking about image. One of the things LA taught me is that, sadly, how you look is often more important than whether you can deliver the goods. I need to bring both to the table.

There's no way around it, anyway. I am a plastic surgeon, trained in Beverly Hills. It's my brand. Says so right here on my card, on my office door, on my website. It's not the Detroit Plastic Surgery Center. It's the *Beverly Hills* Plastic Surgery Center. Even though I may not judge a person by the car he or she drives, others will judge me. Bottom line: driving a shiny new car says something about who you are, and success begets success. That's it.

Oh, one final point.

I hate this car.

It makes me feel like a freaking ramen-eating, Salvation-Army-clothes-wearing student. Or a grown man working a paper route. Or a man-child living in his dad's basement. It embarrasses the crap out of me.

My car issue clutters my mind as I clunk in and out of back roads, the ancient RAV4 wheezing on life support, on my way to give a talk at the home of one of the major donors to Rochester's orchestra guild. I've been invited to discuss "Innovations in Plastic Surgery." Not to be crass, but I'm on a mission. I know my audience. These are well-connected folks, physicians, spouses of physicians, and leaders of the local community who can spread the word that I'm a top-notch doctor to refer people to. Not only that, but they're prime candidates for a little nip here or tuck there. I can't let them think I'm some loser poser who drives a car their unemployed deadbeat teenage grandson wouldn't be caught dead in.

It starts to snow. Fluttery snowflakes waltz by my windshield, no harm, no foul. Suddenly nasty little white spiderweb shapes slap onto the glass right in front of me. I turn on the wipers. They screech and jerk across the windshield like a poor old man who's lost all muscle control, smearing filthy crud across the window, leaving a brown smudge the color of doggie doo. Visibility disappears. Never a good thing when you're, you know, driving. I curse and lean forward, squinting through a crack in the crud, not even as wide as my necktie.

This is not a question of image, or brand, or my desire to look like a raging success. This is now a question of life and death.

"I need a new *car*!" I scream.

Somehow I make out a driveway on my right. I take a shot that I've come to the correct address and turn up what soon becomes a steep hill. The snow whips faster and thicker. The wipers growl and slam ineffectually against the brown crusty splotch rapidly accumulating on the windshield. I slow to a crawl and edge up the hill, the bald tires slipping, causing the RAV4 to skid and stumble like a cartoon drunk. Ahead I make out a mansion and a line of cars (nice cars, I notice in my panic, *really* nice cars) parked in front. I fight to steer clear of their rear ends. I feel my car's tires losing their grip on the driveway and—I can't believe this—the RAV4 grinds and whirs and starts to drift backward like a snowball rolling out of control down the hill.

A car horn blasts behind me. In my rearview mirror, I see a Mercedes gliding up the hill with effortless German precision, warning me to stop driving like an idiot, the driver a matron in a fur coat, gesturing wildly that I'm going in the wrong direction.

"Lady, I know I'm sliding down the hill!" I yell inside my car. I'm pretty sure she can hear me. The Mercedes comes closer and closer. Instinctively, I duck. All I need is for a potential patient to see me, the guest speaker, the guy who's about to present a semi-professional-looking slideshow, pitching her for her business and word-of-mouth, driving not only this piece of crap car but allowing it to plow backward into her gleaming new Mercedes.

I somehow swerve out of the Mercedes's way, allowing it to effortlessly pass me on the right. I let the stupid RAV4 slide downhill until it mercifully conks out unconscious, close to the bottom of the driveway. I turn the ignition back on and allow the RAV4 to complete its coughing jag before it finally turns over. Then I pull to the side of the road as far as I can, hugging the right side of the driveway. I shut off the car, curse for the millionth time, flip up my collar, grab my box of slides, and walk up the hill, trying to hide my face as another five cars pass me on their way up to my talk.

When I finally arrive at the mansion, and after I swill some wine and gobble hors d'oeuvres offered on trays by robotic tuxedoed waiters, I manage to deliver a passionate lecture on what's new and exciting in the world of plastic surgery. I receive great applause and several people promise to phone for a consultation and refer me patients. After some small talk, I walk out of the front door of the mansion feeling satisfied and hopeful.

Then a sheet of snow pelts me in the face. The snowfall is blinding. I spot my RAV4 at the bottom of the hill, about a hundred yards away. I inch down the steep hill in my tasseled wingtip loafers, slipping, sliding, and eventually wiping out on my back, my slides scattered throughout the snow. As I hit the ground, one thought occupies my mind:

I need a new car.

* * *

I keep the cursed car. I have to. Until we make some dent in our debt, I have no choice but to live with the dents and the dings and the disgrace of driving around in that death trap that screams: I'm poor and unsuccessful. When I meet patients at the surgery center where I perform most procedures, I make sure I arrive a half hour earlier so I can park a half mile away from the building. On three occasions, I run late and while I'm climbing out of my RAV4, I see my patients parking and in plain sight. To avoid being seen in or near my total humiliation of a vehicle, I do what any reasonable, rational doctor would do in my situation.

I hide.

The first time I press myself against a tree. The second time I duck behind a UPS truck. The third time I get busted. *Oh, hello there! Luckily, I broke into that old, abandoned car just in time to release a trapped puppy and some orphans. Are you ready for your surgery today?*

* * *

A few days after I perform one of my first procedures, a tummy tuck, my patient shows up at the office. She's in distress. I drop everything and see her immediately.

"I think I might be having a problem," she says.

"You are," I say. "You're bleeding. Nothing to worry about. This happens sometimes, but we need to get you back to surgery."

"OK, like when?"

"Like now. Immediately. I'll meet you in the hospital."

"I can't go."

"Why not?"

"I don't have a car." I stare at her. She must see the sudden shock wave that pulses through me because she explains, "My friend dropped me off."

I'm not proud of this, but all I can think is, *Are you kidding me? You don't have a car? Damn! Damn! Damn!*

"IguessIcandriveyou," I mumble, mashing the entire sentence into one garbled unintelligible glob.

"What? I'm sorry, I didn't understand what you..."

"I'lldriveyou."

She stares, stunned.

"I'll...drive...you," I stammer.

Moments later, we sit silently in my horrifying RAV4 as I jiggle the ignition switch, urging, cajoling, begging the cranky, increasingly noncompliant car to turn over. Finally, the ignition catches and the car lurches forward. In my periphery, I see my patient gripping the sides of the passenger seat, her face going white—from her loss of blood, I tell myself, not from discovering that this is, in fact, the rambling wreck that her esteemed doctor drives.

"So," she says, "this is your car? With a cassette deck and a cracked windshield?"

"No," I say. "I mean, yeah, no, oh, no...*my* car? No. It's not *mine.* I borrowed this from a friend. My...Mer...Beemer...is in the shop."

"Oh."

She sighs and closes her eyes.

She looks relieved.

* * *

My practice picks up, gradually, but I schedule many more consultations than procedures and I have far less money coming in than we need with the months-long wait for insurance payments. I pretty much accept anything that comes my way, the rallying cry of everyone starting out in a new business.

One surgery I do hesitate to accept and then reluctantly agree to perform is called an Asian eyelid operation. In short, I create an extra fold of the eyelid to make a person look "less Asian." In Korea, some mothers opt to have the procedure performed on their daughters because they consider the look more attractive. In Beverly Hills, I watched Dr. Bouley perform the surgery twice and read several articles describing this procedure. Being of Korean descent, I felt both intrigued and a little repulsed by the underlying morality that this surgery implied. Is it so bad to have eyes that look Asian?

Now, several months later, I'm facing this ethical dilemma myself. It's the classic *Sophie's Choice* situation. On the one hand, I don't really believe that making an Asian face look Caucasian is the right thing to do. And the idea that looking like a white person is more attractive than looking Asian pretty much says that my own race is inherently lesser. I really don't want to perpetuate that kind of thinking, especially when it's coming from a mother passing that down to the next generation. But it's my job to give the patient what she wants. And what she wants is an extra fold in her eyelid.

I hesitate, I equivocate, I vacillate. In the end, I reluctantly agree.

* * *

I mark a twenty-five-year-old woman's eyelid in preparation for the surgery in my office as her mom sits across from me and watches. The mom scoots to the edge of her chair and straightens her back.

"Doctor Youn," she says suddenly, the volume of her voice snapping at me like the crack of a whip, rattling me. I nearly fumble my marking pen. "How many these procedures you done before?"

I want to lie.

I want to make up a number that sounds reasonable, a number that suggests I've done enough of them so that the mom and the patient don't have to worry, but not so many that seems illogical, given my age.

"You mean, approximately?" I say.

"Yeah, round number."

"I'd say..." I look up at the ceiling as if I'm trying to recall and calculate the total. I clear my throat and my voice rises into a soprano as I say, "None." I clear my throat again, and my voice sinks into a low register, a deep doctor bass, and I repeat, "Yeah, um, none."

"None?"

"Yes. Zero. That would be the roundest number I could..." And then I speak bullet fast and blurt, "But I have watched two of them and I've read tons about the procedure...."

"OK."

The mom settles back in her chair.

"OK?" I say. "We're going ahead? I can continue marking?"

"Heather, you OK?" the mom says to her daughter.

"I'm cool."

"Great, me too," the mom says. "I wouldn't have anyone else do it."

"Oh, good, yes, then I'm...cool," I add.

The procedure goes well.

Mom and daughter love Heather's new "less Asian"—more Caucasian—look.

I don't. I have a real problem with it.

Why should looking Asian be considered unattractive?

It shouldn't.

Even though I'm desperate for work, I abandon the procedure.

And to this day I've never done another.

* * *

My practice continues to expand.

Slowly.

The massive boost that *Dr. 90210* gave to my burgeoning practice has now slowed to a sputtering trickle. So I continue to hustle, giving local talks, working on my website, and writing letters to other plastic surgeons, offering my help with assisting them in surgery or seeing any patients they don't want to.

I take calls at two of the smaller hospitals in the region. I work on wounds, perform reconstructive surgery, and take emergency room visits. The pay isn't great, but I feel blessed for any work I can get. And then, miraculously, a second hospital—the largest and most respected one in the area—offers me work and privileges. Being on staff at this hospital will give me the credibility and prestige I long for, I need.

I feel as if I've finally arrived. Well, maybe not so much *arrived* as poked the pinky toe of one foot inside the door.

I schedule my first operation at the hospital. I am to perform a breast reduction on a thirty-year-old mother of three. Her breasts have gotten so large and heavy that she suffers from terrible back pain. Previously, during our consultation, my patient arrived with a copy of a Victoria's Secret catalog. Kinda my idea. I suggested she look in magazines or catalogs to see if she could find a model's breasts that approximated the look she wanted to achieve with her surgery. This was a classic Dr. Bouley tactic. Not only would he suggest that patients check out the models in Victoria's Secret, but he kept copies of the catalog in the office for easy reference. During the actual procedure, he would rip the pictures out of the catalog, tape them on the wall of the operating room, and try to match his patient's new breasts to the ones in the photos.

It's not nearly as creepy as it may sound. Although, I don't know, maybe it is. I was in Beverly Hills at the time, and there it seemed perfectly normal. But as I've learned, *normal* means something very different in Beverly Hills than it does in Metro Detroit.

"Hey, yeah...her," my patient says during our consultation, pointing at the catalog. "I want to look like this."

I tear out the pictures of the gorgeous busty model. I too will tape the pictures on the wall of the operating room during the surgery. The photo will become my blueprint.

The day of the procedure, my second day at the hospital, I arrive in the operating room, Victoria's Secret photos in hand. I greet the members of the team who will assist me—the nurse, the scrub tech, and the nurse anesthetist, someone I've not worked with before, a dour-looking woman in her late fifties. I explain about the breast reduction procedure and how I use the Victoria's Secret photos as a guideline, a practice I picked up in Beverly Hills.

"Are you guys OK if I put these pictures up?" I look around the room. I take in a series of nods of approvals and shrugs. "Are you sure you're cool with it?"

Nobody objects.

I tape the Victoria's Secret photos to the wall and refer to them during the surgery. The procedure goes well—no complications, no complaints, little conversation.

That night Amy works late and I decide to celebrate my first successful procedure and my new relationship at the area's best hospital. I hit the Red Lobster and settle in for a long, leisurely meal. I order and lean back, taking in the view of the parking lot, focusing on the horizon. My career—my life—feels different. I feel a shift, the wind finally in my sails. Until now, the wind has been blowing in my face, gusting, full of hail the size of golf balls, forcing me to walk in place as I get pummeled. It's been a struggle—drowning in debt, struggling for what seemed like a decade getting the contractor to complete the office build-out, literally knocking on doors and accosting disdainful strangers with my business cards, desperately trying to round up patients by giving dozens of talks, getting shot down again and again by clinics and other doctors. Until finally I have been accepted at the one hospital in the area that really matters. *Dr. 90210* made people notice me. Getting into this hospital will move me to the next level. *It's a game changer*, I think. *I'm on my way. At last.*

My cell phone rings. I peer at the unfamiliar number, which immediately takes me to a place I call Nervous Town....

Oh, no, a complication from today's surgery.

I picture the worst. Ruptures, bleeding, lawsuits.

I can't help it, that's what I do.

I answer the phone, my voice cracking a little. "Doctor Youn."

"Doctor Youn, this is Susan. I'm the nurse who worked with you today."

I blow out a soft whistle of relief. It will prove to be premature. To say the least. "Oh, yeah, hi, Susan. How are you? What can I do for you?"

She lowers her voice as if she's a spy letting me in on classified information. "I just wanted to warn you that there are some bad things going on."

"Huh?"

My forehead flushes.

A kind of electric shock stabs through my entire body. My stomach starts to rattle and throb. I immediately think of Gina, the Italian model who tried to sue me. I start to sweat. I look down at my plate of food and nausea sweeps through me.

"What...what's going on?" I can barely squeak out the words.

"So, when you put those pictures up in the OR today?"

"Yeah?"

"Apparently the nurse anesthetist was extremely offended. *Extremely*. She's written you up to the Chief of Surgery and she's trying to get you kicked out of the hospital."

I gasp. I can barely breathe.

"Doctor Youn?"

Somehow I manage to say, "I'm here."

Susan continues in a burst. "I'm calling to let you know that I—and the scrub tech—are not offended. Not at all. We were there too, obviously, and we know you asked if it was OK to put up those pictures and nobody said a thing."

"Nobody said a word," I say.

"We understand what you were doing and we think it's perfectly fine. You want your patients to be happy. That's the most important thing. But..."

She drops her voice to a near whisper. "You're in big trouble."

Regurgitation roils in my guts. I place my hand over my mouth and turn away from the food. I look out the window at the parking lot. I turn back and stare at the empty chair opposite me. I turn to my right and look across the dining room. I shift in my chair. I don't know where to turn or where to look. I'm afraid that I really will throw up.

"We're going to stick up for you. I mean, we'll try, if anyone asks us. We're definitely on your side...."

I don't hear anything else she says. Her words pour out without meaning in a low-level buzz, like the whir of a distant chainsaw. At some point, I hear myself saying, "Thank you, I appreciate your support," as if I am some politician running for office. I end the call. I stare straight ahead, the rest of the room blurring.

I'm going to get kicked out of the hospital after two days*? That has to be a freaking record. Wow. I'm amazing.*

I don't sleep that night. My mind is ablaze. I don't think I've done anything wrong. I want to do something to defend myself. But what? I have no idea. Do I write a letter? Do I try to head off the Chief of Surgery? Do I humble myself and apologize, beg the offended nurse to forgive me? I get out of bed and pace. I finally sit at the computer, start to compose my defense, give up, collapse on the couch, and bury my head in my hands.

The next morning the hospital's Chief of Surgery calls me.

"I need to meet with you." His voice trails off ominously. "We have to discuss a situation that has come up. I'm going to get together with you, the Chief of Plastic Surgery, and one of the hospital administrators, the head of the operating rooms. Obviously, this is a serious matter."

I mumble something even I don't hear and, feeling completely impotent, I agree to his first suggested meeting time. I want to deal with this as soon as possible.

"I assume you know what this is about?"

"I do."

"Yes, well, we've received two complaints."

"*Two* complaints?"

"Yes."

It's more serious than I thought.

I don't say that.

I can't.

My throat feels as if it has filled up with sand.

* * *

Five minutes before my meeting with the hospital bigwigs, on my way to the Chief of Surgery's office, I walk through the area next to the OR where I hung the Victoria's Secret photos. I walk with a touch of anger. I laser in on the faces around me. I want to find the second person who turned me in. I know this much: whoever made the second official complaint could not have been in the operating room with me. Yet still they wrote me up. *Who is it?* I think, my head swiveling, glaring, looking from face to face. *Which one of you hates me so much that you want to kick me out of this hospital?* As I walk toward the Chief of Surgery's office, I know I'm projecting, but I feel everyone in the room staring daggers at me.

I knock softly and enter the Chief of Surgery's office. I find what feels like a three-person tribunal waiting for me. The Chief of Plastic Surgery, Dr. Shanahan, a noble-looking man with a shock of salt-and-pepper hair and a bushy salt-and-pepper beard; and Dr. Arruda, a trim woman in her sixties with a boyish haircut, a narrow face, two black lines for lips, and granny glasses hanging on a neck chain, the frames of which she massages absently and constantly. They sit in chairs in front of the Chief of Surgery, Dr. Sizemore, who sits at his formidable desk. Dr. Sizemore is a massive man with a year-round tan and a face that looks chiseled out of granite. He gestures toward an empty chair across from him, between Dr. Arruda and Dr. Shanahan.

"Thanks for coming in, Tony," he says, as if I had a choice. "Please. Sit down."

I nod toward the empty chair. "The hot seat, huh?"

No response.

Dr. Sizemore folds his hands on his desk and leans into me. "Let's get right to it. Doctor Arruda?"

The administrator in charge of operating rooms fiddles with the frames of her glasses and crosses her legs. She wears a blue pinstriped business suit and what looks like a pair of men's dress shoes.

"OK then," she says, gesturing with her glasses. "So, you've been written up for this. This particular person is very upset and is threatening to accuse you of sexual harassment."

I lose it. "*What?* Sexual *harassment*? I didn't harass anybody, sexually or otherwise. I asked everybody in that operating room if they were OK with my putting up the pictures. Nobody said a thing. If anybody had an issue, I would've been happy to take down the pictures. Or if they said something in the beginning, I never would've put the pictures up."

I take a deep breath, embarrassed by my verbal spewing.

"I'm sorry for the outburst," I say. "It's just so..."

I can't finish the sentence. *I'm dead.* That's all I know. I look at Dr. Arruda, seated tautly, severely, her expression all ice and fire. I glance across at Dr. Sizemore, his tan, Mount Rushmore face nodding. He looks like a judge about to slam down a gavel proclaiming a guilty verdict, sentencing the accused to a lifetime of hard labor in a Siberian gulag. Or, in my case, banishment from this hospital. Forever.

Silence descends and the room seems to go dark.

Finally, Dr. Shanahan, the Chief of Plastic Surgery, speaks.

"Well," he says in a deep, bass voice, sounding like a radio announcer. "This is complete bullshit. We have to throw this out. And what is she talking about? Sexual harassment? That's a load of crap. Get rid of that. It's garbage."

"Yeah," Dr. Sizemore, the Chief of Surgery says. "Tony, you're a nice guy and here you are, on your, what, second day, and you have to deal with this? Don't worry about it. We'll take care of it."

Dr. Arruda clears her throat and pops the tip of her frames into the corner of her mouth. Dr. Shanahan takes her cue.

"Doctor Arruda?"

"Yes, I have a definite opinion as well."

Here it comes, I think, the dissenting opinion that will get me expelled from this hospital for life, derailing my career, just when it was finally getting off the ground.

"Please," Dr. Sizemore says, waving at her to speak.

"I believe that the complainant, based on what I've seen, heard, and read...has a stick up her butt."

I think the others laugh, but I don't really hear them because I'm too busy saying, "Oh, my God, thank you. Thank you so much. I've been such a wreck over this. I never meant to offend anybody."

"We know," Dr. Sizemore says. "It was unfortunate that you got this pile of dog crap dumped on you."

"And so soon," Dr. Shanahan says.

"Took the rest of us much longer," Dr. Arruda says.

Now I join them in their merry laughter. The energy in the room crackles with *joie de vivre*. The dark light dissolves. Suddenly all is right again.

"I just want to do the right thing," I say. "I want to develop a good reputation, take care of my patients well, and be a productive doctor in this hospital."

"Oh, you'll be fine," Dr. Shanahan says. "I have no doubt."

"Thanks again for coming in," Dr. Sizemore says. "Hope you didn't lose any sleep over this."

"I slept like a baby. I was up every two hours."

It's an old, bad joke, but they laugh as if they've heard it for the first time.

I walk out of the Chief of Surgery's office and wander back through the hospital with my head held high.

19

"Look at Me!"

All is well. Or so it seems. The threat of being branded a sexual harasser has gone away, a ridiculous blip, and my status at the hospital seems more secure every day, but I still can't sleep. I know that I'm a good doctor. I know, even more, that I *care*. Of course, I want to make a living and pull myself out of debt, but making money does not drive me. I know it sounds like a cliché, but I really want to help people. That is my reason.

And then something happens that nearly destroys me.

* * *

I see a patient for a consultation, a woman in her midfifties, a former model, she claims. I will call her Madame X. She caught my appearance on *Dr. 90210* and has sought me out. Madame X tells Hannah, my receptionist, that she needs to see me immediately. Hannah fits her in that afternoon. "You're from Beverly Hills," she says during our consultation. "You're the only doctor who can help me. I'm sure you are so much better than anyone in Michigan."

"I don't know about that," I say.

"Modest. I like that. But I know better. Did you not train in Beverly Hills?"

"I did. I spent a year...."

"Say no more." She sighs sadly. "Look at me. I've had all this botched work done. You're the only one who can fix it."

As I examine her, I see an attractive woman who looks like she's had a few operations. I notice some mildly thickened scars from a previous facelift, a few small indentations in her cheeks, and some jowls and loose skin under her neck. I think, *I don't see anything too bad. She doesn't look botched. Overall, she looks pretty good, but with a few minor tweaks maybe I could help her feel a little better about herself.*

"OK, so what did you have in mind?" I lean against my desk, folding my arms.

Madame X answers with the fluency of a medical colleague. "As you can see, I still have some jowls and these hollows under my eyes. I was hoping you could inject some fat and maybe redo my facelift. And could you maybe do a brow lift?"

I look her over. "Yeah, I think that's reasonable. We can do that."

She sniffs. "I'm very unhappy with this last result. The doctor who did my surgery wasn't even a real plastic surgeon. I found out later he was a fake. Not board certified. A total quack. I was taken in and botched. Can you believe it?" Her voice catches, and she stares at the ground.

"I'm really sorry to hear that," I say. "I can't guarantee you that I can make you happy, but I will promise you I'll do my best."

"The whole thing has been a horrible ordeal for me and my family. It's been so upsetting that...that...I've missed out on job promotions because of how bad I feel about myself. I even took out a loan for ten thousand dollars to pay for the surgery. I paid him ten thousand dollars and now he refuses to take my calls or fix what he's done. How could I pick such a horrible doctor?

How could I have been so stupid?" She looks up at me with pleading eyes.

I hold her hand in both of mine. I feel bad for her. I really do. "I'm so sorry you've been through all of this. I'll tell you what. Let me chat with my office manager and see if I can do most of this pro bono for you. Maybe we can take a really bad thing and make something good out of it."

Her eyes water. I think she might cry.

"Doctor Youn," she says after composing herself, "you are my savior. I don't know what to say. Thank you."

"You're welcome. I just want you to be happy." I feel good that I can hopefully help this poor woman get her life and self-esteem back on track.

* * *

I perform Madame X's surgery. Everything goes smoothly. A week later, she returns for a routine follow-up. She looks puffy, which is normal and expected, but otherwise she's recovering nicely and on time. She returns in three weeks for her second follow-up. She's still puffy, again expected, but otherwise progressing perfectly. And she seems happy. Satisfied. Hannah schedules her next follow-up appointment in another three weeks.

Madame X calls the office a week before her appointment. She's panicked and she's decidedly *un*happy. Hannah puts her right through to me.

"There's something terribly wrong," Madame X says. Her voice goes flat and cold as steel. "I need to get everything fixed."

The same wave of nausea that fluttered through my stomach when I learned there was a sexual harassment complaint about the Victoria's Secret photos grips me again. Only this time I not only feel like heaving, I start to sweat.

"What's wrong?" I ask Madame X, trying not to sound as panicked as I feel.

"Everything is wrong. I'm in severe pain and my face looks terrible. You ruined me. You need to refer me to some other doctors who can fix what you destroyed."

"Look, OK, I want to reassure you. It hasn't even been six weeks. We really need to give it more time to heal completely. But how's this? Why don't you come in..."

"I'm not coming in until I see at least one other doctor."

I pause. I'm on the verge of hyperventilation, and I need a moment to catch my breath. I swallow audibly. I wipe my sweaty palms on my pants, and say, "I'll get you a name. And after you see him, come see me and we'll talk everything through. We'll figure this out together. How does that sound?" I wait for her response. I hear her breathing. Then I hear the dial tone. Madame X has hung up on me.

I call Dr. Shanahan, the Chief of Plastic Surgery at the hospital I now attend more regularly. After his support in the meeting with the Chief of Surgery, we've struck up a good relationship. And his noble salt-and-pepperiness always makes me feel better. I explain the situation with Madame X. He's incredibly accommodating, agreeing to see her the next day. Hannah arranges the appointment.

The day of her scheduled six-week follow-up with me, Madame X blows like a low-pressure front through the waiting room into my office. She's furious. "I saw Doctor Shanahan, as you suggested. And do you know what he said? He said that I'm a *train wreck* and there's absolutely nothing he can do to fix your incompetence."

My mouth drops open like a trapdoor.

There's no way he said that. He would've told me if he thought I'd botched the surgery. Plus, no doubt about it, she looks pretty good.

"I'll check in with him, but frankly I'm surprised he said that," I say. "Because you look fine. You really do. First, remember, you're only six weeks out. Your brows look good. Your neck is nice and tight. Your scars are healing well. I honestly think it's just a matter of a little more time. Here are some creams to apply to your scars. On the house. If it's OK with you, let's have you come back in two weeks and reassess then."

She snatches the tubes and jars of cream, stuffs them into her purse, sneers, "I'll be back," and storms out of the office.

I turn into an eyeball-popping, noneating, barely functioning, high-voltage, nerve-ending insomniac. I know that Madame X is a ticking bomb about to explode. And when she does, she's going to explode all over me. The only questions are where and when and how?

One evening Amy and I take a long walk and discuss potential scenarios, including the one in which Madame X sues me, buries us financially, and ruins me forever. I decide to anticipate this. I call my malpractice company. The woman I speak to offers me a possible escape route.

"Return her money and make sure she signs a release," she says. "I'll fax you the form."

The day of Madame X's next appointment, I fill out the release form and pull out my checkbook. I write her a check for more than the amount that I charged her for the surgery. I don't care that I'm losing a ton of money on her. I want this unstable ticking time bomb out of my life, out of my head, and out of my nightmares. I tear out the check and put it in my pocket. A few minutes before Madame X's appointment, I warn Hannah that the woman is not only angry, she's possibly explosive.

"Oh, I'm aware," Hannah says, "which is why I scheduled her as your last appointment. I don't want her freaking out and scaring a waiting room full of patients."

I thank my lucky stars for Hannah.

"That would be a fun scene, wouldn't it?"

"I should get combat pay." She gives me a wry smile and for just a second, I feel better.

I thank my lucky stars for Hannah again.

I retreat to my office and wait.

I don't wait long.

I hear the outer door bang open.

Madame X bursts through the waiting room, a human tornado. "I need to see Doctor Youn! I need to see him *now*!"

She charges into my office, her still slightly puffy face aflame with rage. She grips herself across her midsection and screams, zero to sixty in a millisecond, roaring, "You messed me *up*! You botched *everything*!"

I try to calm her, go into my most soothing bedside-manner voice. "I really think you look fine. In fact, since I knew you were coming in, I talked with Doctor Shanahan and asked him what he thought of your results and if I did anything wrong. He said, 'No. She looks good. It's a nice result.'"

Madame X doesn't hear me. She's too deep into diva screeching mode. "*You botched it!* I have so much searing pain in my cheeks from where you took that knife and *dug it all through the inside of my* face."

She narrows her eyes to slits and drops her voice an octave, speaking now with horror movie menace, becoming Vincent Price in a dress. "You should know this pain. I should let you know how this feels. You want to know how I feel, Doctor Youn? I feel like my face went through a windshield. Yeah. That's what I should do. I should slam your face through a windshield."

I lose control of my eyelids and blink at her rapidly. "Are you threatening to hit me with your *car*?"

Madame X growls. "I'm in a lot of *pain*."

I nod, force myself to stop blinking like I'm part of a REM experiment. "OK, I understand. Now, let's please settle down. I get that you're in pain...."

"You don't get it. You don't get it at all. You have no idea how I feel. My face is on fire. You took that massive knife and you just kept stabbing me in my face, stabbing me, stabbing me, stabbing me. And now look at me. What kind of doctor are you? Are you even licensed? Look. At. Me. I'm *hideous!*"

It's not easy, but I force a smile. "It was just your ordinary standard-issue scalpel and honestly, I swear, you don't look hideous, at all."

"You made me look *Oriental*. You made me look like *you.*"

OK.

It's official.

She has BDD.

Body dysmorphic disorder.

The psychiatric condition where a person's self-image is completely out of line with reality.

Many doctors suspected Michael Jackson of having BDD.

They are also the patients most likely to murder their plastic surgeon.

What the hell do I do now?

"I really don't know what to say to that," I say. "But for the record, I promise, you don't look Asian."

Then Madame X reaches a whole new level of intensity. She starts crying, blubbering uncontrollably, her deafening wails cutting like foghorns through the building.

"You've ruined me, you've ruined my life, you've cost me two job promotions, and now I have to get all of this fixed and I can't afford any of it. *Look at me!*"

"I see you. I really do. You're swollen, still, but that's it. Please listen to me."

"I'm *hideous.* And I'm going to *destroy you.*"

Her weeping skids to a stop. She looks at me as if noticing me for the first time.

"I want a million dollars," she says.

"A mil...OK, listen..."

"If you don't pay me one million dollars, I will sue you for everything you have. I will destroy your life and your career. I will make destroying you my mission, my entire goal in life. I will make it the *air I breathe*. I'm going to make you crawl all the way back to Beverly Hills on your *knees*. I will make it so that the only people who will ever allow you to operate on them are the whores!"

"The...what?"

"The *whores*! The *whores*! The *whores*!"

She sprints out of my office, arms flailing, high heels clopping. I dash after her. She's staring into the full-length mirror mounted on the wall in the waiting room.

"*Look at me!*" she bellows at the top of her lungs. I'm afraid the sonic waves blasting out of her mouth will shatter the mirror into a million shards. "I'm a hideous *monster*!!!"

I glance frantically around the room. I catch a glimpse of the top of Hannah's head bobbing behind the front desk.

"Please," I say, my voice calm, cool, measured. "Come back into my office and let's talk this out."

Madame X pivots toward me and I swear I see smoke pouring out of her nostrils. "You're all talk, aren't you? The smug Beverly Hills doctor is all *talk*. I want one million dollars, Doctor Smug. One million dollars and not a penny less or I will bury you."

I take a deep breath and exhale slowly. "You're not getting a million dollars. I don't have that kind of money. I don't have anything close to a million dollars."

She draws herself up and locks herself into a frozen tableau. "Give me a hundred fifty thousand. I'll take a hundred fifty thousand."

Great. Now I'm playing *Let's Make a Deal* with Medusa.

"I don't have that kind of money either."

Madame X punches her hands against her hips and gives me the once-over like I'm a car she's about to buy. "Then give me *carte blanche*. For the next two years, you pay for anything I want done by any other surgeon I choose, anywhere in the world. I want *carte blanche* for two years."

"I'm sorry, I can't do that. It's not possible." I take a step closer to her and, finding my most reasonable tone, I pat my pocket. "I have a check here for more than what you paid me for your surgery." I sidestep to the front desk and grab the release form lying on the blotter. I offer it to her. "If you sign this release form, the check is yours. But that's it. We're done. Sign the release form and I'll give you the check. You'll make a nice profit off of everything that has happened between us. In essence, I will have paid you to perform your surgery."

Her bottom lip trembles. She raises her index finger to the ceiling, then points it at the floor, and then jabs it in my face. "Do you think you can buy me off for less than *a hundred and fifty grand*? Are you insane? I'm not one of your whores. I'm going to destroy you. I'm very connected in this town and I will drag your reputation through the dirt and mud and you will never have another patient and you will run away from here, *run away,* like the disgusting little smug maggot you are. *More than what I paid you?* You insult me. I will never take that money."

Her head thrown back, she stomps out of the office and slams the door behind her.

It's suddenly blessedly quiet. I hold for a beat and then turn toward the front desk. "She's gone. You can come out now."

Hannah slowly appears from behind the front desk. "Oh, my *God*! That was not in my job description."

"Mine either."

"I thought she was going to kill us. What if she comes back with a gun?"

"She's not gonna come back with a gun."

"Just in case." Hannah runs to the front door and double locks it.

"It's gonna be fine," I squeak. I try to sound convincing. I don't even come close. The nausea snakes slither back into my gut.

I breathe heavily, close my eyes, and stand in the waiting room, my world spinning. My knees buckle like a building being razed, and I lean onto the side of the couch beneath the full-length mirror, to stop from keeling over.

"Are you OK, Tony?"

"I'm fine," I say, trying not to heave. I repeat, moronically, "Everything's gonna be just fine."

"You know I was kidding about the combat pay...."

I mutter again that everything's gonna be just fine, force a feeble grin, and stagger back into my office. I take a couple of slow, shallow breaths, sip from a bottle of water, and say aloud to the room, "My God, what the hell am I going to do?"

I stare at my cell phone. An idea pops into my head. I pick my phone up and within seconds I'm frantically dialing the one person I know who's been in this position, at least once, with an angry, disgruntled patient who actually stalked him.

I call Dr. Romeo Bouley.

I get right through to him and in one long barely incoherent rant I fill him in on my experience with Madame X.

"Wow, yeah, been *there*," he says. "I feel you, Tony."

"She's nuts. She's screaming at me, threatening me. I'm afraid for my life."

"Oh, I know. Same thing happened to me. This woman followed me. I'd see her everywhere. I'd look out the window of my house and see her in the bushes. She'd stay there all night. I'd look out in the morning and she'd still be there, staring at me. It was creepy as hell."

"What did you do?"

"Simple. I hired a couple of guys to beat her up."

My head feels like it's spinning around on my neck. I grasp for the arms of my desk chair and sit heavily. "You *what*?"

"Yeah. I asked around, found a couple of people who do, like, *contract work*, you know? They beat her up. Took care of everything. Never heard from her again. Cost a few bucks but it was worth it. I'm sure you can find guys in Detroit who'd be happy to help you out. Just tell them you want the *Good Fellas* special."

I start kneading the bridge of my nose. "I can't do that."

"Well, it's a thought."

I hear pounding on the front door.

Wham. Wham. Wham.

"Oh, my God. She's back. I wouldn't be surprised if she has a gun."

"Call the cops."

"I have to go."

"Let me know what happens. This is great."

Great? Not the word I would use.

I hang up the phone and run into the waiting room. Hannah squats behind her desk, gesturing wildly at the door. Her face has gone white.

Wham.

Wham.

Wham.

I feel like a man in a horror movie. I spread myself against the wall and slink inch by inch toward the front door. I duck and look out the window. Sure enough, it's Madame X. She pounds on the door again. I look carefully and see no sign of a gun. I reach over and unlock the front door.

Madame X storms into the waiting room, rushes right by me, blasts to the front desk, grabs a pen, scribbles her name on the release form, picks up the check on the blotter, and stuffs it into her purse.

"You can come out now," she hisses at Hannah, who crouches behind the front desk, her arms covering her head.

Madame X walks right up to me, puts her face inches from mine, and glowers and hisses like a serpent. "This is not over."

She brushes past me, strides out the open front door, and slams it behind her.

"She's gone," I say.

A long moment passes. Finally, still crouched under her desk, Hannah squeaks, "I need a drink."

* * *

After Hannah leaves for the night, I phone three friends, plastic surgeons, and ask them if they've ever had dealings with a patient like Madame X. None of them have.

And then, in a moment of weakness, or madness, or pure sadism, I call my residency archrival, the immortal Doctor Garth Ellington, Superstar, already one of Miami's new crown prince plastic surgeons. After an awkward few minutes of hello, how-are-you, catching-up chatter, I pop the question. "Have you ever had a patient flip out on you?"

"What do you mean?"

"You perform a procedure and even though it goes well, she doesn't see it? In fact, she's so upset and hates what you've done so much that she threatens to destroy you, literally destroy you. This woman threatened to run me over with her *car*. For starters."

"Wow," Garth says. I can hear his voice go cold. I should've never called him. "No. I've never had anything like that happen to me. Never."

"You've never had an unhappy patient, someone who wanted her money back...."

"Oh, no. All my patients have been very happy. I had one patient who was so happy she wanted to pay me *more*...."

I realize this is the last person I should be talking to, so I pretend I have another call coming in and hang up before he can finish.

* * *

I burn with doubt.

I ache with fear.

I quiver with uncertainty.

I clutch the covers and flip over in bed for the hundredth time and face the digital alarm clock on my nightstand.

2:14 a.m.

The numbers mock me.

The last time I checked it was 2:12 a.m.

I came to bed at 11 p.m. I have not slept one single blink.

Next to me, her sleep my envy, Amy rumbles softly.

My eyes wider than they've ever been, I stare at the shadows on the ceiling.

Next morning—well, *this* morning, in a few hours—I will perform the longest and most complicated operation of my so-called career, a five-hour reconstructive surgery for a breast cancer survivor.

The fever of my doubt soaks me in the sweat of the damned.

Should I even be doing this?

Am I in the right field?

Maybe Madame X was right.

Maybe I did ruin her.

Maybe I have no skill.

Maybe I don't belong here.

Maybe I should just quit.

* * *

Six a.m. I roll out of bed. I call my patient.

"Megan, this is Doctor Youn," I say. "I hope I didn't wake you."

"No, no, that's all right."

I shut my eyes as I speak into the phone. "I'm really sorry, but...I don't think I can do your surgery."

"What?" She sounds upset, alarmed, anxious. And who can blame her? "Why?"

"Something happened yesterday and...I just don't think I can do it."

"OK, well, that's fine, so let's reschedule...."

"No, you don't understand," I say. "I don't think I can *do* it. Ever. You need to find another doctor."

"Really? This is so..."

"I'll refund all your copays and deductibles and I'll refer you to a plastic surgeon who will do a better job than I can. I'm so sorry about this."

My eyes still closed, I slowly hang up the phone.

* * *

I cancel all my consultations for the next morning. I can't see anyone. I envision a parade of kind, cooperative, respectful, prospective patients who abruptly turn into a mob of hissing, shrieking lunatics who threaten me, fists in the air, and then sue me, attack me, and bash my head in with thick folders of legal documents. Then I see myself in my scrubs, mask on, about to begin a surgery. I freeze, holding my scalpel aloft, sure that I'll botch the procedure and leave the patient a horrible mess. I drop the scalpel, back away from the operating table, tear off my scrubs and mask, and run out of the room.

I'm being irrational, I tell myself. *I'm letting one completely irrational, unreasonable patient crush my confidence*. I understand that intellectually. Emotionally, I don't feel capable of getting through even a simple consultation.

I spend the afternoon at the hospital rounding on patients. I go through the motions, halfheartedly making notes on charts, answering questions with generic answers, nodding dumbly as nurses and patients speak to me, their sentences a nonsensical garble.

Late that afternoon, I get into my car in the hospital parking lot knowing that I'm suffering from exhaustion and extreme stress. I prescribe myself a decent meal, a quiet night with Amy, and a good night's sleep. Despite feeling shaky and on edge, I vow to man up and return to my practice in the morning rejuvenated. Before I exit the parking lot, my cell phone rings. Hannah. I pull over and take the call.

"What's up?" I ask, my voice a low monotone.

"You know our favorite patient?"

"What now?"

"Her mom just called. She says she needs to talk to you right away." Hannah pauses, waits for me to respond. When I don't, she says, "The mom said her daughter is suicidal."

"Oh, no," I say. "I'll be right there."

Driving the twenty minutes from the hospital to my office, a terrifying mixture of thoughts clutters my mind. Beginning with utter disbelief that this woman is actually going to take her life. First and foremost, I pray to God that she doesn't hurt herself. She clearly is in distress and needs the kind of care I can't provide—the psychiatric kind. But how *can* I help her? She obviously despises me and blames me for everything. And if I can't stop her, how can I live with one of my patients committing suicide because of me? Did I really cause her life to become unlivable? What kind of physician am I that my patient wants to kill herself because of what I did?

This last, final thought shatters me:

I may have to give up being a doctor.

This could be it, the end of my career, the end of the line. When word gets out that my patient committed suicide after going under my knife, my practice, all that I have spent my life trying to build, will be destroyed. No one will want me as their doctor.

What will I do? I'm not trained to do anything else. I have no other skills. Will I have to become a cabdriver, a server, a salesclerk?

Will I apply for a job at Best Buy selling electronics? Or maybe become a greeter at Home Depot? Will Amy leave me?

Madame X got her wish. She's ruined me.

By the time I arrive at my office, I'm a complete wreck. Hannah hands me a slip of paper with the mom's number. I grab it, my hands shaking, the paper fluttering, go into my office, and close the door. I study the phone number for a few seconds. I dial a different number instead, my friend Tim, my closest pal from medical school, a psychiatrist now at Michigan State University College of Human Medicine. I tell him the saga of Madame X, her homicidal threats, how she ultimately signed the release and grabbed my check. I end with the punch line—her mom's calling me because the daughter is now suicidal. Tim listens patiently, attentively. When I pause to breathe, he says, "Is that everything?"

"Yeah. What do I do? Do I call her back?"

"Yes, you have to." Tim speaks with urgency. "You call the mom back and tell her to contact the police immediately. Tony, you don't have a relationship with the daughter anymore. She signed the release and that ended it. She's no longer your patient. You should not contact the daughter yourself. But you have to tell the mother to call the police right away and get her daughter and bring her to a hospital. It's definitely serious."

"OK, I will."

"One more thing. Write down when you called the mother, write down the whole conversation. You should document the whole thing, everything your patient did, right from the beginning."

"All right. Thanks, man. I'm gonna call the mom now."

"Call me back if you need anything and let me know what happens."

"I will."

I call Madame X's mom. She picks up on the first ring as if she's waiting for my call.

"This is Doctor Youn returning your call." I try to extinguish the wildfire of pulsing anxiety raging inside me.

"Oh, yes, Doctor *Youn*. My daughter told me all about *you*."

"I got your message and I'm very concerned."

"You should be."

"You need to call the police, right away."

She hesitates. "The police?"

"Yes, absolutely. If your daughter is suicidal, you need to call the police and have them pick her up and bring her to the hospital. We don't want anything bad to happen to her."

"Oh," the mom says. I think I hear her laughing. "She's not suicidal."

I hold for a beat. "She's not?"

"No. That was just a figure of speech. She's not going to kill herself. That's crazy."

I tap my forehead with my cell phone. "It's...crazy?"

"Yes. She just needs more money to take care of all the botched work you did. You need to pay her more."

My mouth opens, closes, opens, locks shut, blocking my ability to speak. Finally, I unclamp my lips and I say, "Are you *freaking kidding me*?"

The mom says nothing.

"I want to make sure I understand this," I say. "Your daughter asked you—her *mother*—to call me to shake me down for more money? Or was this your idea?"

"You're being very disrespectful. I'm eighty-five years old, I live alone, and I'm in failing health. I have a weak heart. Too much stress and I could drop dead at any minute."

I want to say, *Fine, drop dead,* but instead I manage to say, "If your daughter is suicidal, you need to call the police. Period. The end. This conversation is over."

I hang up the phone.

Suddenly I feel better than I have in days.

20

Psychiatrist with a Scalpel

Aftershock.

That's what I feel.

During consultations, I scrutinize every potential patient, assessing what they want me to do with less than my full attention, most of my focus locked in trying to look under their skin, into their soul, to determine if they contain strains of latent BDD or some other psychiatric condition that will bring torment and trauma into my life. Since my debacle with Madame X, I have equipped my internal warning mechanism with a hypersensitive hair trigger, allowing it to bleat inside my head like an overeager high-volume fire alarm whenever I sniff out the slightest hint of BDD or patients who may turn on me.

Then I do the worst thing a doctor can do. I let the fear affect my decision making. I practice overly defensive medicine. I take no chances. I reject, on average, one out of every three patients. Not because they don't need my help. Or because I can't help them. Because I'm scared.

My hypervigilance guts my practice. Less than six months in business, I can't afford to turn people away. But the ghost of Madame X spooks me. I live in fear of people flipping out in my office and of certified letters arriving at my door or process servers ambushing me at the hospital or jumping out from behind a plant at Red Lobster and slapping documents of impending lawsuits against my chest. I look suspiciously at the people who parade into my office eager to have me perform plastic surgery on them and half the time their faces morph into the furious visage of Madame X. My confidence, recently shaken to its core, has essentially gone missing.

It feels like my practice is getting flooded with patients who aren't good surgical candidates. Patients who need a psychiatrist more than a plastic surgeon. My own personal Murphy's Law. I try to weed them out but they multiply instead.

* * *

I meet with a woman whose chart says she works as a librarian in Detroit. I invite her to sit down. She takes a seat in front of my desk and leans forward. She has long hair and rimless glasses. I don't want to get ahead of myself, but she looks nice and unassuming.

"What can I do for you?" I ask.

"Can't you tell?"

The alarm shrieks in my head. But for some reason, I choose to ignore the mind-bending wailing that's honking like a horn in my skull. I shift uncomfortably in my chair. "Um, no, I'm sorry, but I'm not sure what..."

"I see you looking at me," the librarian says. "The way they all look at me."

"I..." I stare at her now, lost. "What do you mean, the way they all look at you? I'm not sure what you're talking about exactly...."

She jabs herself on both sides of her head and screams, "My eyes! My eyes! My eyes! They stare at my eyes! Look at them! They're awful!"

OK, I hear the alarm now. Blaring. Red alert!

I wish I could slink past her or dive out the window.

"Honestly," I say. "I really don't know what you're talking about."

The nice librarian suddenly looks like a killer from a Stephen King movie as she hisses, "Oh, I see you staring at my eyes just like the rest of them. They all come into the library, all of them, students, faculty, city residents, even homeless people, and they all just stare at my eyes. You can see why. They're awful. You need to fix them."

For some stupid reason, I ignore the bells and whistles and alarms screaming in my skull. I don't flee. I continue the consultation.

I move in and look at her eyes. It can't hurt to give her the benefit of the doubt. Maybe there really *is* something wrong with her eyes.

Nope.

Completely normal.

"I see a little bit of extra skin there," I say, "but your eyes really don't look bad...."

"Don't patronize me," she snarls. "You know they're awful. Now, you tell me. What are you going to do for them?"

"I actually am not going to do anything for them."

She doesn't hear me. She barrels on. "I want a price. Give me a price. How much?"

"I really don't..."

"Give me a price to fix my eyes!"

I realize that this is a job for a psychiatrist, not a plastic surgeon. There's no way I'm going to convince her that her eyes are, in fact, just fine. So how do I turn her down for surgery? Without her going off the deep end?

I have a blinding flash of inspiration. I'll use the same excuse that dozens of women used on me back in college when they wanted to turn *me* down and get rid of me. I've heard the line more times than I'd like to admit.

"It's not you, it's me. I'm just not ready or good enough to perform your operation."

Works like a charm.

* * *

Then there's Edith.

A woman in her forties, flabby, her arms fleshy, her face puffy, ruddy, full, her eyes wide and wild, her lipstick smeared, her hair looking as if she'd just walked through a windstorm, her voice loud and gravelly, channeling Linda Blair in *The Exorcist*.

My internal alarm blares the moment I see her enter my office, but even then, it's too late.

"What can I do for you?" I ask, getting a creepy feeling just looking at her.

She wastes no time. She starts ranting immediately. "I almost got beat up in a bar last night because of you!"

"Because of me?"

"Not *you*! Because of people like you. Because of my *plastic surgery*."

"OK, calm down, take it easy. Tell me what happened."

"I had a tummy tuck done, right? About a month and a half ago. And my plastic surgeon..." Edith starts pacing my office like an animal in a cage. "Ooh, I could kill him! If he walked in that door right now, I would kill him. I would rip him apart with my bare hands!"

"I can see you're upset," I say, master of the obvious. "So, tell me, calm as you can, what did he do?"

"I told you! He gave me a tummy tuck!"

"OK..."

"And he left me with a *scrotum*."

"A...? Beg your pardon? Not sure I heard you correctly. Did you say...?"

"Yes! A *scrotum*. He gave me a scrotum. A ball sack."

"Huh?" I say, all other words failing me.

Edith stops pacing and crash lands into the chair next to the examining table. She seems exhausted. "I went on this diet and I lost a hundred pounds and all of a sudden I had all this extra skin. Six weeks ago this *doctor* did this tummy tuck, flattened my tummy. But he left me with this sagging skin off my vagina. It's all sagging." She leans forward and loses it again. "It's all *sagging*! It looks like a big scrotum. A big hairy *scrotum* hanging off of my vagina!"

"That does sound unattractive," I admit. "Just a guess, but a big hairy scrotum is probably not what your doctor was going for. Or what you would want. Have you spoken to your plastic surgeon about this?"

"Of course. He tells me it's just fine and that I need to wait six months before he can do anything else. *Six months?* Are you serious? I can't wait six months. I'm clinically depressed. Because of this I'm going to a shrink. I'm beside myself. I went out to a bar last night with one of my friends and three guys thought I was a transvestite because of the bulge in my pants. They tried to beat me up."

"Maybe you should stay away from bars...."

"Did you hear me? They tried to beat me up!"

"I heard you."

"You have to fix me because he's not gonna do it."

"Well, to be fair, it is normal to wait awhile for the swelling to come down after this procedure. Six months is entirely reasonable."

Edith starts pacing, waving her hands frantically as she speaks. "You know what I did? I hired an attorney. Oh, yeah. I already hired an *attorney*. He can't refuse to fix me. I will *make* him fix me."

I have to get her out of here.

That's the one and only thought in my head.

"Unless," she says.

She glares at me with tiny squinting eyes.

How do these people find me?

"Unless?" I squeak.

"Unless you can fix me now." She pauses, holding her intense stare. "You fix me now, you remove my big hairy scrotum, and I will go away. Forever."

An opening.

An exit strategy.

I have to take it.

"Well," I say, my voice hitting a pitch high enough to shatter glass. "Why don't I take a peek? But I'm telling you, it's not unusual to wait awhile before anything can be done."

"Take a peek," Edith says, batting her eyes. "Why don't you?"

She changes into a gown and I bring in Hannah. Standard procedure when I examine a woman patient. And with Edith, I know I can't be too cautious. I'd examine her from another room, if I could.

Edith lies down on the examining table and I lift her gown and look at her pubic area and I see...

"A *scrotum,*" Edith shouts. "A big hairy scrotum! Look at it!"

I wouldn't call it a scrotum exactly, but next to her recently flattened tummy sits a wad of extra hanging skin creating, yes, a sort of...bulge.

"I see what you mean," I say. "There's some extra skin that's kind of drooping down over there. Uh-huh. And it's definitely still swollen."

Edith lifts herself onto her elbows. "Now what are you gonna do about it?"

"I can't do anything for another six weeks, maybe two months. We have to allow the swelling to go down."

"So, in other words, nothing."

"I can't. You have to wait. It's too soon."

She sits up, fixes that stare on me again, swings her legs off the examination table, and lands on the floor in a kind of ninja crouch.

"That won't do," she says.

"I'm sorry. It'll have to."

"No. If you won't fix me, I'll do it myself."

I frown. "I'm not sure I..."

She gets right into my face. "I'm gonna take a scalpel and cut off my scrotum right now, right here, in your office, in front of everybody."

"Ha-*ha,*" I laugh. "That's funny."

"You think I'm *joking*?" Edith takes a beat and then lunges past me and pulls open a drawer containing medical supplies.

"Hey hey hey! Stay out of there!" I say, shutting the drawer.

She gets back into my face. "Then fix me now...*or I will do it myself!*"

DIY plastic surgery.

I shudder at the thought.

Get her out of here.

Get her out.

I go for a Hail Mary. "I really think it's best to wait until all the swelling comes down but...but I suppose we can schedule a tentative date to do it."

She lifts an eyebrow. "When?"

"Well, let's see," I say, stalling, pretending to calculate.

"When will you *cut off my scrotum*?"

"In four weeks?" I say quickly, hoping, praying that she doesn't want to wait.

"That's insane," Edith says. "Apart from my original surgeon, you're the only one who wants to wait that long. That's way longer than anyone else in the area. And I've seen fifteen other plastic surgeons."

"You've seen *fifteen* other doctors?"

"Yeah. They all said the same thing. They'd operate on me within a week or two."

"Is there anyone you haven't seen?"

"Doctor Shanahan. He's next on my list. He's the only one left."

"He's a good friend of mine," I say. "He's really good. You should see him."

Sorry, Shanny.

"Two months is crazy," she says, gathering up her stuff, preparing to leave. "*You're* crazy."

"Maybe, but there's a lot of swelling and it's a scrotum, kind of unusual for a woman..."

"I know!"

"OK, well, good luck, and I'm sorry if I didn't say what you wanted to hear. Sometimes it's best to get other opinions if you and I aren't on the same page," I say, trying to slide past her.

Edith cuts me off. "Doctor Youn, this has been a colossal waste of my time. Beverly Hills plastic surgeon? Whatever. You're way overrated."

She storms out the door.

I never hear from Edith again.

* * *

One day, a few weeks later, after rounding on patients at the hospital, I bump into Dr. Shanahan. I rather sheepishly bring up Edith, not mentioning names, wondering if she ever called him from my referral.

"Oh, yes," he says. "Scrotum Lady. She was *different*."

"You're not kidding. What did you tell her?"

"Oh, I fixed her up. I did it right there and then. Snip, snip, snip. She's happy. No more ball sack. Thanks for the referral."

"Any time," I say, in shock.

* * *

Some patients present fascinating stories but just aren't candidates for surgery.

I see a young man in his midtwenties who brings his dad with him for our consultation. The young man, thin, pasty, with an uncombed mass of flyaway black hair, scruffy black beard, and wearing a flannel shirt and jeans, holds a large manila envelope. He sports tinted glasses. The dad, sixties, white unruly hair, white patchy beard, wearing a sport jacket over his faded flannel shirt and baggy jeans, stands next to him, rigid as a statue.

"How can I help you?" I say.

"I broke my eye socket," the young man says.

"OK, well, can you take off your glasses? Let's have a look."

He slowly, gingerly, removes his glasses, revealing an ugly black eye.

"You got a shiner, all right," I say. "How'd that happen?"

"The devil did it," he says.

I look at him, then at his father, who doesn't move a muscle.

"Um, what?" I say.

"It was Satan. Satan struck me."

"Satan struck you?" I hear myself say.

The young man nods furiously. "I was at church and I was singing and all of a sudden I felt something hit me flush in the face, like a...a...thunderbolt or...something. Struck me right in the eye. I knew right away it was Satan. Wham! Black eye from Satan. I went to the emergency room and they did a CT scan and it showed right there on that scan that my eye socket was broken."

I nod along with him. "Are you sure something else didn't hit you in the face? Some kind of foreign object or..."

"No, sir," the dad says in a deep, sweet, and insistent baritone. "I was there. We were singing together. All of a sudden something hit him, something you could not see, and my boy fell to the ground. It was Satan. No other explanation. There was nothing else there. Nothing. And nobody. No other person. Nobody else was there. I heard this loud *smack*...."

The dad claps his hands loudly and violently, scaring the crap out of me so much that I nearly leap out of my white coat.

"He *fell*," the dad roars, and then whispers, "It was Satan."

I compose myself and nod at the manila envelope the son holds. "Is that the CT scan?"

"Yes, sir," the son says.

"May I?"

The son hands me the envelope. I pull out the CT scan and pin it up on my viewer.

"Well," I say pointing at the image of his eye socket. "It's definitely broken. But it looks like a hairline fracture. Good news. You don't need surgery."

The son and dad heave simultaneous sighs of relief.

"I'm going to give you some painkillers and put you on a liquid diet for two weeks," I say to the son. "Sometimes chewing can cause the break to get worse, even a slight one like this. Definitely want to avoid that."

I unclasp the CT scan from the viewer and take one final look before handing it back to the son. "You got lucky. Looks like you got punched pretty hard."

"Yes, sir," the dad says. "Satan has a mean left hook."

PART EIGHT

MAKING IT

21

Holding Hands

My business has hit rock bottom. I know financially I need to perform more surgeries to build my practice, but I find I prefer escaping to the hospital, answering calls, tending to emergency room patients, and performing tiny procedures (like mole removals) as ways to boost my confidence, which remains stuck in the gutter.

One day I get a call from Devon, the PA (physician's assistant) who works with Dr. Melrose, a cardiac surgeon. I don't know Devon, but I've met Dr. Melrose a couple of times. He's tall, trim, proud of his ramrod posture, and arrogant as hell. Basically, he's a surgeon who acts like a puffy peacock swashbuckler. I always get the impression when I see him in the hospital that he considers me a bottom feeder several dozen rungs below him in the doctor food chain.

"We have a patient here," Devon says to me on the phone. "She's eighty years old and she just had open heart surgery. We think her sternum may be infected."

"I'm happy to take a look," I say.

I meet Devon in the ICU and examine Dr. Melrose's patient, whom I'll call Helen. In open heart surgery, the cardiac surgeon will saw the sternum in half to gain access to the heart. After the surgery, the surgeon will then put the breastbone back, wiring it together to keep it in place. Sometimes this doesn't hold and a gap forms. The plastic surgeon then gets called in to move muscles from the chest and abdomen to seal the gap, which, hopefully, will allow the sternum to heal. This follow-up operation can be painstaking and delicate and long, often lasting several hours.

In this case, I check Helen and discover that she indeed has a sternal dehiscence, which can be every bit as nasty as it sounds. Her breastbone has split open, and the wires keeping the sternum in place have unraveled. Puss seeps through the opening, infecting the bone, turning it to jelly. In technical terms, we doctors call this result a freaking mess.

I tell Devon the PA what I see and offer to call Dr. Melrose directly. Dr. Melrose answers his cell on the sixth ring and when he does, he sounds annoyed, as if my calling about his patient who's in distress has caused him a monumental inconvenience, and may cause him to miss his tee time at the local country club.

"Hi, Doctor Melrose. This is Doctor Youn. I'm the plastic surgeon on call and I'm consulting about your patient, Helen...."

"Yeah, just take care of that, will you?"

"Sure, of course. Is there anything you can tell me about the patient?"

"She's old."

"Uh-huh. Anything else that might be..."

"How should I know? Talk to the PA. I'll look in on her at rounds tomorrow."

He clicks off in a huff.

I smile at Devon. "Nice guy."

Devon doesn't smile back.

I operate on Helen that night. I remove her dead sternum and perform three muscle transfers. I work slowly, precisely, and meticulously. The operation takes close to six hours. The surgery goes smoothly. I finish at four o'clock in the morning feeling exhausted and exhilarated.

Despite her age, Helen heals well. For the next month, I pop into the ICU and check on her every day. I see slow, steady improvement, her muscles getting stronger, her color and strength returning. This is just the sort of result that makes being a plastic surgeon so rewarding, where I can actually see my patient's life get better on an almost daily basis, as a direct result of my work. I'm reminded why I decided to enter this field so many years ago.

At the beginning of her fifth week in the hospital, she's moved out of the ICU and onto the floor. Always a good sign. I continue to check on her daily.

One night, about six weeks into her recovery, I get stuck at the office working late. I look at the time and realize that I won't be able to get to the hospital until after ten o'clock. I decide to skip this one day and round on Helen first thing in the morning.

I get to the hospital early, before seven, and find that Helen is not in her room. Concerned, I look her up in the computer. My heart sinks. She's been moved back to the ICU.

As I head over to the ICU, an all too familiar *rat-tat-tat* rapid fire of negativity assaults me.

Crap. I miss one day and she ends up in the ICU. What could've happened to her? If only I hadn't missed that one day....

My mind abandons that totally irrational line of thinking and hops right into the murky depths of the worst-case scenario.

Oh, no. Something happened with my surgery. It must be my fault. The muscles I transferred probably came apart. I must've screwed up.

I pick up my pace, break into a near run, fly around the corner, and nearly crash into Helen's family. I introduce myself to the first person I see, her grandson, I presume.

"What happened?" I ask him.

"She had a heart attack last night," he sighs, clearly crestfallen.

"Oh, no, that's horrible," I say.

I feel a tiny wave of relief. Of this I am not proud.

At least this has nothing to do with me. Thank God it's not my fault.

And then in the midst of my seemingly never-ending crisis of confidence I override that thought and go back to—*Wait a minute. Am I sure I didn't do something to cause this?*

I look at poor Helen, hooked up to a ventilator, and peek at her chest. My work seems intact, and healing perfectly. Composed now, shaking off my stupid, irrational, self-hating line of thinking, I slide into total professional doctor mode and ask Helen's grandson, "How bad was it? What did the doctor say?"

"Really bad," the grandson says. "He doesn't think she's going to survive."

"Oh, no," I say again. I look back at Helen, sedated, motionless, a tangle of wires hooked up to seemingly every inch of her, her breaths regular and mechanical, in time with the ventilator. She looks like she's sliding toward death. "I'm really sorry."

He nods, fights back tears.

"I'll keep following up on her," I say. "There's nothing I can really do at this point. But I promise to check in on her."

"That would be great," the grandson says. "But I don't want you to think you have to...."

"I want to," I say, looking down at this woman I've poured so much of myself into. "She's my patient."

I spend a few more minutes with the family and then seek out Dr. Melrose, the cardiac surgeon. I find him strutting down the corridor, his posture strong, his beak of a nose pointed toward Heaven, his excellent hair sculpted and gelled. He speaks into the air, a scribe nipping at his heels like a puppy, frantically taking notes.

"Excuse me, Doctor Melrose," I say, catching up to him.

He stops in his tracks, blinks at me in confusion. Like he's never seen me, even though I'm the doctor he brought in to, you know, fix his patient. "Can I help you?"

"I'm Doctor Youn," I say, introducing myself to him for probably the tenth time.

"The plastic surgeon?" I add when he looks at me with a blank face, pretending he's never met me.

"Oh. Yes?"

"I wanted to ask you what's going on with Helen, the patient I operated on a few weeks ago, who went into cardiac arrest last night...."

"Talk to the PA." He dismisses me with a condescending wave, as if I'm the help, turning back to dictating notes to his eager, sycophantic scribe.

I stand alone in the corridor, seething, watching this jerk playing God.

* * *

I check on Helen the next day.

She lies comatose, attached to the ventilator, her eyes closed, her breathing rhythmic, sounding artificial and metallic. I feel helpless, hopeless, lost, knowing there is nothing I can do for her. I pull a chair next to her bed and, purely by instinct, grab her hand. Her fingers feel cold and nearly lifeless. I gently fold my fingers over hers and hold her hand in mine for five or six minutes. I keep my head bowed. When I'm not consciously praying, I focus on trying to connect to Helen. Mainly, though, I simply try to *be*. With her.

I come back the next day and hold her hand again.

And I come the next day. And the next. And every day for a week. Each day I hold Helen's hand. She, of course, doesn't know it, since she isn't really conscious or awake. Still, I sit with her and hold her hand.

About ten days later, when I come into her room, she seems in a state approaching consciousness. I'm not sure what makes me think that. All signs, every bit of information I receive from her family and from the PA Devon, indicate that she is falling deeper into unconsciousness and that she is not going to survive. But something about her today makes me challenge that. When I look closely I can see that her color seems better. Her eyelids flutter. I pull the chair over to her bed and sit down. When I do, she reaches out her hand to me.

I take her hand and hold it. This time I say, "Hey, Helen, how you doing? I think you're getting better. Hang in there, OK? I'll be back tomorrow."

The next day when I come in she again reaches for my hand. I continue to check in on her every morning, hold her hand, and talk to her with soft encouragement.

One morning I come in and Helen is sitting up in bed, off the ventilator, breathing on her own.

"Holy cow, Helen," I say. "Look at you."

She smiles widely. "Guess I'm not dead yet."

"I guess not," I say. "Everybody wrote you off. But you're still here."

She looks in my eyes. "Really? Everybody gave up on me?"

"Well, maybe not everybody." I smile. "But I mean it. You're a miracle."

She shrugs. "Miracles happen."

"Unbelievable. Everything looks great. You're healing fine. I think you're gonna make it, Helen."

I pull the chair close to her bed.

"I want to tell you something, Doctor Youn," she says.

"What's that?"

"I knew."

I must look confused because Helen pushes herself forward a little and says with quiet urgency, "I knew that you came in every day and held my hand. That made a big difference. I looked forward to seeing you every day. I just want to say thank you."

"I was just doing my job," I say.

Helen reaches over and takes my hand.

"No," she says. "This was beyond your job. You weren't doing your job. You were being kind. I will always be grateful. You saved me."

She squeezes my hand. I smile at her.

"In a lot of ways, you saved me too." I squeeze her hand in return.

I continue to check on Helen for the next two weeks until her doctor releases her from the hospital. A few days after she's home, a bouquet of flowers so big it would put the winner of the Kentucky Derby to shame arrives at my office door.

The card reads: "Doctor Youn. Thank you forever, Helen."

22

Thrown Under the Bus

Helen's recovery gives me a new lease on life and boosts my confidence—temporarily. But I'm soon cut off at the knees again. This time I'm blindsided by an appalling incident at Helen's hospital, the home of conceited and coldhearted Dr. Melrose. A place I'll call St. Nowhere.

One Friday at around five o'clock I receive a call from a physical therapist. She asks if I will come to her office immediately and see a patient who's recovering from knee replacement surgery. I drive to the office, which is close by, and examine a woman in her sixties, whom I'll call Jane. Jane had her knee replaced two months ago and it still has not healed.

"What's going on with it?" I ask her.

"Sorry to be graphic," she says, "but I've got an open sore that keeps leaking pus."

"That's not good. An open wound leaking pus is never good. You say it's been two months?"

"A little longer, actually."

"That's really not good," I say, shaking my head.

"What's happening with it?"

"My first thought is the joint could be infected. If that's the case, your orthopedic surgeon will have to take out the prosthetic he put in. You can't clear up the infection with an antibiotic or even surgery."

"So he might have to remove my knee replacement?" she asks, eyes opening wide.

"Yeah, unfortunately, if it's infected it has to come out. I'm happy to call him and talk about it." I pat the top of her hand.

She agrees, so I do.

I call her orthopedic surgeon, Dr. Blackheart, whose haughtiness through the phone simply *reeks.* He couldn't appear more annoyed or put out. What is it with the surgeons at this hospital? Do they all aspire to be Dr. House? I explain that I've just examined his patient Jane and suggest that her knee joint may be infected.

"Impossible," Dr. Blackheart says.

"Well, with all due respect, I'm a little concerned that the joint has been dripping pus for more than two months, aren't you?"

"No, I'm not. The joint is fine. Do you know *how* I know it's fine?"

"Ah, no."

"I know it's fine because I did the work. I only do good work and therefore the joint is fine."

I'm not sure how to respond to this level of blatant arrogance and ego. I don't have to because Dr. Blackheart tells me what I will do since I've been brought in by *his* patient.

"Now that we've established that the joint is fine, I think you should move a muscle over. I would suggest a calf muscle. The muscle will take care of the minor infection."

"OK," I say, my pulse pounding, my confidence deflating like a tire with a spike stabbed through the tread. I fight to keep my balance, to stand my ground, to advocate for the patient with pus oozing from her knee.

"But here's the thing," I finally say. "I don't think moving the muscle is going to help because the muscle is probably going to just pus out. If the prosthetic is infected, it won't heal, no matter what I do with the muscle."

"I'm fully aware of that, Doctor Youn." He sighs mightily, acting like I'm King of the Village Idiots. "I have been doing this for twenty-five years. I know that the *joint is fine.* When you've been in practice as long as I have, you know these things, as you, yourself, may possibly learn some day. Right now you need to move a muscle over the knee. Can you or can you not do that for me?"

I'm boiling, my forehead aflame. My voice cracks as I say, "I'm happy to do it for you. No big deal."

"Thank you," Dr. Blackheart says, sounding as if he actually said, *Screw you,* and then he hangs up.

* * *

A few days later, I operate on Jane's knee. I move a flap from her calf muscle and place it over the infected area of her knee. I honestly hope that Dr. Blackheart's diagnosis is correct. I hope that the new muscle will bring in a new blood supply and clear out the infection. The operation takes three hours and goes without a hitch.

Four days after the surgery, I check in on Jane. She's healing well.

"You look good," I say to her.

"Yeah, I think it's coming along," she says.

"I'd say you're getting close. Probably be going home soon."

"Oh, I'd love that."

"Are you having much pain?" I ask her.

"No, I'm notttttarghrowwww," she says, and her eyes slam shut.

"Jane?"

She doesn't seem to hear me. She looks...gone.

"Jane! Are you OK? *Jane!* Can you hear me?"

Nothing.

"Jane!"

She doesn't respond.

I race out of the room and run toward the nurses' station.

"Call a code!" I scream. *"Call a code!"*

I skid to a stop, turn around, and hear the nurse calling a code through the loudspeaker overhead as I rush back into Jane's room. I pull up at her bedside, grab her wrist, and take her pulse. I'm in full-blown life-or-death emergency mode, my own heart pounding. I hold my breath and then blow out a whoosh of air. Her heart is beating and she's still breathing.

"Jane!" I say, my face close to hers. "Can you *hear* me? Answer me."

She doesn't react. Her face seems petrified. Her breathing comes slower and shallower.

"Code!" I shout again.

Then a commotion at the door, rubber wheels banging the doorframe as a nurse curses low and pushes in a crash cart. She hooks Jane to a heart monitor and from the crash cart I grab a manual resuscitator, a gas mask, place it over Jane's face, and force feed her oxygen.

Time freezes.

I feel my arm tremble.

My mind flashes through snapshots of medical school, residency, and working in the ER, and I realize I haven't taken care of a patient who is coding in probably four years. My thoughts race. But then sense memory clicks in and I'm holding the gas mask in place and watching Jane breathe—I'm *bagging* her—and I'm glued to the heart monitor. Suddenly her eyes flutter and open into slits.

"Jane," I say. "Are you OK?"

She manages a nod.

I remove the mask.

Her eyes pop open wide and she says, quietly, "What happened?"

"I don't know," I say. "You were unresponsive."

"I don't remember..."

As she speaks, I see that she's moving only half her mouth. Her other half has drooped like a large jowl.

Not good.

"I think you've had a stroke," I say. "I'll be right back."

I put the mask back over Jane's face to keep her breathing steady. I nod to the crash cart nurse to take over. I walk past another nurse who's hanging back, on alert, it seems.

"Where's the hospital physician?" I ask her. "Isn't there a house officer here?"

"Yes," she says, following me into the hall. "He's on this floor."

"Because, see, I'm a plastic surgeon and if this woman's having a stroke, you don't necessarily want a plastic surgeon taking care of her."

"Already paged him," she says, giving me a look that I can't read. On cue, a short, trim Asian doctor in white scrubs rounds a corner and strides toward us. He wears heavy sensible shoes that clomp on the slick hospital floor. As he walks, he flings his arms violently in front of him, as if he's a private in a Far East army. I'm afraid he'll march right past me.

"Yes?" he says, stopping short and looking up at me. I'm a head taller at least. He blinks insanely. "I am health officer Doctor Park. Who are you?"

"I'm Doctor Youn. Tony. Tony Youn."

He blinks—he doesn't stop blinking—turns away, turns back, his blinking causing me to start blinking.

"Do you have something in your eye?" I say.

"New contacts," he says. "Pains in my *butt*. They make me *cry*."

"I'm sorry. Listen. I think this woman just had a stroke. She's starting to come out of it. She's breathing fine now. Her heart's fine. But I think we need to send her to the ICU and have a neurologist look at her. And probably an intensivist too. Do you feel comfortable taking care of this? I'm a plastic surgeon and this isn't really my expertise."

"Oh, yes, *yes*. I take care of it. I definitely take care of it."

Blink*ing*.

Despite my best efforts not to, I find myself blinking back.

"Is there anything you can do about that?"

"Oh, yes, I *know*. Excuse *me*." He turns away, leans over, and pops his contacts out into his palm. He slips them into his coat pocket.

"There," Dr. Park says. "Much better. I can *see*."

He tilts his head back, looks up at me again, his eyes wide, red, and watery. "Yes?" he says.

"Well," I say. "Should we check on the patient?"

"Yes. Oh, *yes*."

He grins and doesn't move a muscle. I take the lead and walk into Jane's room, Dr. Park folowing, practically climbing up my back.

"That's her," I say, pointing to Jane in the bed.

"I *know*."

He doesn't move. I wait for him to do something—anything—and when he makes no attempt to step in, I say, "Do you think you should take the mask off?"

He shoots me a sheepish grin. "Oh, oh, OK, yes, I take it *off*."

Hands flying in front of him, nearly spearing the nurse working the crash cart in the ribs, he arrives at Jane's side and grins down at her. "I am Doctor Park," he says. "I am here now."

"I'm going to call the family," I say. "They need to know what's going on."

"Oh, yeah, good, you do that, OK," Dr. Park says.

I go back out to the nurses' station and find the same nurse who paged Dr. Park. "I need to call the family," I say. "Can you get me an outside line?"

Her face darkens. "Where's Doctor Park?"

"He's in there. With Jane."

She looks stricken. "What? You left him alone with her?"

"Well, he's the house officer, right? Isn't he the overnight doctor?"

"I guess. I mean, yeah."

The nurse turns away, pretends to shuffle through some paperwork.

"What's the matter?" I say. "Isn't he supposed to take care of emergencies?"

"I don't know."

"What are you talking about? What does he do?"

She fixes me with a freaked out, five-alarm look. "Basically, the only time we call him is when we need him to order Tylenol for people."

I feel as if I've entered a lost episode of the *Twilight Zone*. "You get him to give you Tylenol? Is he even a doctor?"

"I think so," the nurse says.

"A doctor of what? What's he a doctor *of*?"

"I have no idea," the nurse says.

I bolt back into Jane's room. Dr. Park stands over her, the mask still in place over her face. He hasn't moved since I left.

"Doctor Park," I say.

"Yes?"

"What are your plans here? Are you sending her to the ICU?"

"Do you think we should?"

"I think so. Yes."

"OK."

I stare down at him. He fixes me with his stupefied grin. I wait.

"Do you think we should call neurology and an intensivist?" I say, finally.

A head tilt. More blinking, despite his contacts now resting comfortably in his pocket. "Do you think we should?"

"Yes, I do, yes."

"OK. Yeah. Let's."

My head pounding, I hold for a count of three. I study the floor, scanning past Dr. Park's disturbingly stupid grin, and then bring my head up, stare into his wide, red, watery, and probably nearly blind eyes, and say, "Do you feel confident taking care of her?"

"Oh, yes, yes, sure, *yes.*"

Again, the grin, and I laser stare at him and I think...no, I *know*...

This guy has absolutely no idea what he's doing. He is completely clueless.

"Do you want me to just go ahead and take care of this right now?" I say in a rush.

"Oh, yes, yes, that would be *fine*."

"OK."

I nod at Dr. Park, who steps back, bows, and gestures as if he's allowing me to cut in front of him in a checkout line at a grocery store. I slide past him and remove the mask from Jane's face. She's breathing regularly now and the shape of her mouth has returned to normal, half of it no longer droopy and immobile. I lean over and speak softly. "Jane, are you breathing OK?"

"I am. I'm feeling all right."

"OK, good. I think you've had a stroke, maybe a TIA."

Her eyes cloud over in confusion.

"That stands for transient ischemic attack, a mini stroke. We're going to send you to the ICU to check everything out, make sure that's all it is."

"All right," she says.

I can see that she's rapidly coming out of what I'm more and more convinced is a TIA. I leave her in the care of the nurse, Dr. Park hanging back against the wall, focusing his attention now on what appears to be a recent manicure. I go back out to the nurses' station and call the intensivist, who happens to be rounding in the hospital. Within minutes, she arrives, a take-charge, tall Asian woman, who frowns when she sees Dr. Park backing out of Jane's room. She murmurs something I'm not meant to hear, but I'm fairly certain she says, "God help us," before she reviews Jane's vitals with me and the details of what will in fact turn out to be a TIA.

Jane stays in the ICU for a couple of days and then returns to a room on the floor. I visit her every day, monitor her progress. On the third or fourth day, as I do during each of my visits, I check her knee. This time the incision has opened up and pus is leaking out.

In this instance, I hate to be right.

"Oh, man," I say, trying not to show my impatience or annoyance.

"What's going on with my knee?"

"The muscle looks fine. But you're still leaking pus. I really think your joint is infected. You need to talk to your orthopedic surgeon about taking out the prosthetic."

She doesn't look happy. Like she'd rather live without a knee than confront Dr. Blackheart.

"I'll write a note for Doctor Blackheart on your chart," I say.

I take her chart out of the sleeve attached to her door, walk to the nurses' station, and write, "Knee has begun draining purulent material again. Concerned it may be from the joint prosthesis. Muscle flap appears viable. Await orthopedic surgery input regarding possible infection of prosthetic. I will continue to monitor from a plastic surgery standpoint. No other plastic surgery recommendations at this time."

I come back the next morning and before I go into Jane's room, I slide her chart out of the sleeve on the door. Dr. Blackheart has responded to my notation on her chart. In blue ink so bold you can feel the anger scream off the page, he's written, "The joint is fine. Need a second opinion from another plastic surgeon. The muscle flap has failed. *Muscle flap has failed.*"

I seethe. I swallow a strong urge to scream and slam my fist into the door. I take a deep breath, exhale, and enter Jane's room, plastering on a fake Dr. Park smile. After checking her over, I call my friend, the plastic surgeon Dr. Shanahan. I ask him to look at Jane.

Two hours later he calls me.

"Tony, your muscle flap is fine. That knee is full of pus. The prosthetic has to be changed out. He needs to take care of this."

"Thanks. Did you write that on the chart?"

"I did."

That afternoon I receive a call from Dr. Blackheart. Bracing myself, I answer my phone as casually as I can. "Hello? This is Doctor Youn."

He begins speaking in a roar and builds. "Who the hell do you think you are telling me that *my knee joint is infected*?"

I pause, more to catch my breath than to allow him to cool down.

"Look," I say. "I'm not the only one who thinks the joint is infected. The other plastic surgeon thinks so too."

"Are you an orthopedic surgeon?"

"What does that...?"

"Are you an orthopedic surgeon?"

I say nothing.

"Are you an orthopedic surgeon?"

"No," I say.

"Then you know *nothing about orthopedic surgery.*"

I clench my teeth. "That muscle is fine. She's had pus coming out of that joint for three months. There's only one logical explanation. It's the joint."

His voice goes thin and cold. "You don't know what you're talking about. I'm going to get another plastic surgeon to take a look at her."

"You want a *third* plastic surgeon?"

"That's right."

"Fine. Go for it. I have no problem with that. But why don't we get a second orthopedic surgeon to look at her too?"

He flips out. "Never! I will never do that! Are you telling me that I don't know what I'm doing?"

"No." I'm proud of how calm I keep my voice. "I'm saying that it's in the patient's best interest to get another opinion from an orthopedic surgeon as long as you're getting another opinion from a plastic surgeon. You're having three plastic surgeons look at her. Why not have two orthopedic surgeons? What's the harm?"

"You know what? This is your fault. I'm telling the patient that this is all your fault. Your muscle flap failed. That's why she's infected. I'm going to get a new plastic surgeon, a different plastic surgeon, somebody *good.* I don't need you taking care of her anymore. You're done."

He hangs up on me.

I'm tired, I'm furious, I'm emotional.

I want to throw my phone against the wall.

Instead, I leave the office early and go for a long, hard run.

To sweat out my fury.

That night, still angry, my head throbbing, I toss and turn, not getting more than an hour total of sleep.

In the morning, I see Jane for what I know will be the last time.

I assume she's up to speed on Dr. Blackheart's diagnosis, his opinion of me, and his insistence that I'm the moron responsible for the infection in her knee—even though she had the infection before I first examined her.

"So, I saw my orthopedic surgeon yesterday," she says. She lowers her eyes and puffs out a half smile. "He says this is all your fault."

"I know. We spoke yesterday. We don't see eye to eye."

"Apparently."

"You realize that you had the infection months before you saw me, right?"

"I know. I honestly don't understand why he's blaming it on you."

"That makes two of us. I can only guess. Maybe because I'm young, I'm new, and he's the expert. In any case, I'm stepping away. But I urge you to see another orthopedic surgeon. If he's going to bring in a third plastic surgeon, why not go for a second opinion from an independent orthopedic surgeon?"

She shrugs.

"It's your call," I say. "It's your knee."

She laughs and shrugs again.

"So, I guess this is good-bye. I really wish you well, Jane."

She reaches over and grabs my hand. "If it weren't for you, when I had that stroke..."

Now it's my turn to shrug.

And then Jane says, "I know it's not your fault. He may be blaming you, but I'm not."

"Thanks. That means a lot." I press her hand in both of mine, wish her well again, head back to my office, and try to not think about Jane and all the doctors I recently dealt with at that hospital—Dr. Blackheart, Dr. Park, and Dr. Melrose, a veritable potpourri of incompetents and arrogant pricks.

About six weeks after Dr. Blackheart dismisses me from working with Jane, Hannah knocks on my door.

"You really have to see this," she says, looking solemn.

"What's the matter?" I say, that too familiar sour taste of impending doom rising into my throat.

She winks and I trail her into the waiting room.

A massive gift-wrapped package overwhelms the coffee table. I consider it for half a second before I rip into the crinkly wrapping paper and find...an assortment of *pies*—blueberry, apple, cherry, pecan, rhubarb—enough pies for a month of Thanksgivings. I grab the ornate envelope speared into the center of the sparkly cellophane wrapping paper. I tear it open and read: "Doctor Youn. Thank you for taking such good care of me. No doctor has ever given me so much time and attention. You truly are the best. I didn't bake these pies, although I could have now that my knee is so much better. Thank you again, Jane."

I laugh and my heart soars. I distribute the pies among my staff, and then call Jane to thank her and to find out what happened with her knee.

"Quite a story," she says. "So, after you left, my doctor had another plastic surgeon see me. Number three. Older man. He basically stood in the doorway and looked at me from across the room. He said, 'Why don't we just keep an eye on this for awhile?' And then he left."

"That was it?" I say. "That's all he did?"

"Yep. He didn't inspect my knee or anything. Just kind of glanced at it from a distance. I didn't want to say anything, but he seemed kind of checked out."

"Seems so," I say, thankful that Jane can't see me shaking my head and mouthing *jerk* through the phone.

"So, then, finally, I got to go home, but my knee kept draining and draining and draining. At last, about three weeks ago, my orthopedic surgeon examined me and said he had to replace the joint because it was infected."

I try to disguise my growl of disgust.

"And how are you now?"

"Doing much better. The infection is gone and I'm walking. I go to physical therapy three times a week. Coming along nicely. I'm going to be fine."

"All I can say is I'm glad to hear it."

"And I want to say thank you again for taking such good care of me and I'm sorry you had to go through so much...*garbage.*"

"These things happen," I say, thinking, *These things seem to happen to me, like all the time, especially at this hospital.*

I'm truly touched by Jane's gift and tell her so before we hang up.

* * *

That night, after everyone else leaves, I sit alone in my office. I pull up a chair and look out the window, watching darkness come, my hands folded in my lap. I think about the past twelve months since I've begun my practice—dealing with the trauma and subsequent fallout from Madame X and then the consistently awful treatment of both me and my patients at one of the regional hospitals where I have privileges. In Jane's case, if I hadn't taken over when she suffered her mini stroke—well, I can't go there. I just know that she wouldn't have been given adequate care. In addition, we both had to deal with the arrogant and egotistical Dr. Blackheart, who, after nearly four months, finally, reluctantly, removed an obviously infected prosthetic from her knee. He acted as if he were on the payroll of the company that manufactured the implant. I later found out he was.

I kick the chair away from the window, stand, and peer into the dark, moonless night, losing myself in thought. I make two decisions.

Decision number one: First thing in the morning, I drop my privileges at the hospital. I'll be strangled financially, with no steady income flow, just money trickling in sporadically. Especially if I continue to sift out so many of my cosmetic patients. I don't care. I will not admit my patients to a hospital where I don't feel they'll be safe.

Decision number two: I'm taking Amy to Jamaica.

23

Jamaica, Say You Will

I need to get away.

I long to veg out on a beach, soak up some rays, swim in a cool blue ocean, gorge myself at an all-you-can-eat buffet, get a massage, and clear my head.

Michigan in winter can have its own charms, allegedly, but this winter, with my ego feeling crushed like a grape, my nerves hot-wired and jittery, and my Spidey sense's continuous tingling, I need to chill. Amy, feeling fatigued and stressed at work—well, in fairness, because of me, she might be feeling stressed at home too—also needs a break and a change of scenery.

We trawl the internet and land on a spot that at least online takes our breath away. A gorgeous resort in Jamaica. We ask people we know who've been to Jamaica and everyone gives the place two thumbs up. And, they say, if we're patient and conscientious, we can find plenty of super deals, especially if we pay upfront. I am nothing if not patient and conscientious. I really want to take Amy to Jamaica. Living with me this last year, she's definitely earned it.

We find the perfect place, a resort that offers a week of luxury, gorgeous beaches, beautiful pools, incredible food, wonderful partying, and super-friendly people.

We book it.

Our confirmation email pings a few seconds later.

"Congratulations and welcome," the email reads. "Now prepare for an unforgettable week of *Hedonism*."

"Hedonism?" I say, frowning at Amy. "What exactly does that mean?"

She scratches her temple, frowns back. "OK, you know what moderation means? Abstinence? Self-restraint?"

"Sure."

"Those are not hedonism."

* * *

I love the resort.

Our room is amazing—a king bed with soft sheets and puffy pillows, a large bathroom with a walk-in shower, and a view of the blue ocean lapping up onto sand white as talcum. In no hurry, we lounge around the room for awhile, trolling through the free-movie channels, and then head down for dinner. We scan the restaurant for other hedonists but don't see anyone who looks the part or who's even close to our age. We go back to the room after dinner and decide to put on our bathing suits and scope out the rest of the resort, maybe hang out in one of the "amazing, soothing, sensual hot tubs," according to the glossy brochure we find peeking out from under the telephone shaped like a conch shell on our night table.

An hour after dinner, Amy, wearing a sporty bikini, and I, tucking a couple of towels under my arm and wearing a Jimmy Buffet cargo-style swimsuit and a Hawaiian shirt, stroll past a peanut-shaped outdoor swimming pool. Nothing unusual about this pool except that it's deserted, not a soul around. We keep walking and arrive at a second pool. Clusters of people sit along the perimeter talking, feet dangling into the water, and a few others catch an evening swim. This pool features a stunning waterslide in the middle that rises as high as a two-story building and, ridiculously, at the far end, a trapeze.

"Interesting," Amy says, hands on hips, scouring the area like she's a cop on *CSI Jamaica*.

"Very," I say. "Are you sure *hedonism* doesn't mean fun in the circus?"

"Possibly," Amy says in this tiny voice that I've learned indicates, *Watch out, trouble ahead,* which I hate because she's always right.

We scoot past the circus pool, turn a corner, and arrive at a secluded, deserted, bubbling hot tub.

In other words, paradise.

"Now this is what *I'm* talking about, Willis," I say, laying down our towels.

"Oh, yeah," Amy says.

Holding hands, we tiptoe into the hot tub. The hot water rises and seeps into my pores and almost instantly my mood changes. Every toxic cell in my body, every poisonous encounter, every negative sense memory that has been stored up from the past few months is drowned by the warm, bubbling purity of this water. Calm falls over me, washed away with a torrent of my sweat. Before I close my eyes I tilt my head back and look up into the night. I feel engulfed by countless stars descending like a light, tropical snowfall.

"I may be in heaven," I say, closing my eyes.

"Those stars," Amy murmurs.

"I want to stay here forever," I say. "Just the two of us."

"Hmm, hmm," Amy says and leans in for a kiss.

"Mind if I join you?"

Booming voice.

Scaring the crap out of me.

A mountain of water swamps me like a wave as a buck-naked fifty-five-year-old fat guy with a bald head, bulbous belly, and a carpet of hair covering his entire body cannonballs into the hot tub, his basketball-sized scrotum hairy as a toupee jiggling inches from my face.

"You don't *mind,* do you?" he roars.

"Ha, hi," I say.

"I'm Mel," bald hairy naked guy says, extending a gorilla paw in my direction.

"I'm...Jerry," I say, looking at Amy, whose eyes have gone huge with horror. "And this is Lu..."

"Carla..." Amy says.

"LuCarlotta," I say.

"Pleased to meet you both," Mel says, flashing a fence of yellow teeth with intermittent gaps wide enough to floss with a jump rope. "This your first time here at Swingers Week?"

"Swingers Week?" I say, hoping I haven't just shouted.

"Yep," Mel roars. "All you can eat for the week, clothing optional. As in, pack light. As in, nudity not required, just heavily suggested."

He widens his grin and leers at Amy.

"Hedonism," I whisper to Amy. "I think I just figured out what it means."

"What?"

"Perverts in paradise."

"This is my seventh Swingers Week," Mel says. "In a row. Seven in a *row.* Never left unsatisfied. Always come back for more."

Another leer at Amy and this time he adds an attractive eyebrow wiggle.

"So," Mel says, "where is the lovely couple from?"

We stare at him for ten seconds.

"Minnesota," I say, finally.

"Minneapolis," Amy says.

"St. Paul," I say at the same time.

"The Minneapolis-St. Paul *area,*" I say. "A little town. You never heard of it."

"Might have," Mel says. "Got family there. Try me."

Amy and I look at each other.

"Mamasanlollapaloozaville," I say.

"Don't know it," Mel says. "What line you in?"

"I'm a doc..."

Amy elbows me in the gut, hard.

"...umentary filmmaker," I gasp.

"That is fascinating," Mel says. "I love show business."

"Aspiring," Amy says. "He's an aspiring documentary filmmaker. Right now he's just, well, we're just..."

"Brokers," I say. "Real estate brokers. We broker real estate. Boring."

"I hear you," Mel says. "I sell insurance. Also boring. And that's why we're here, right? To lose ourselves in the heat of the moment?"

Another leer at Amy and this time he drools.

"Speaking of heat," I say. "It sure is warm in here. I think we're going to get out and cool off. Shall we, LuCarlotta?"

"Sure...Jerry."

As I help Amy out of the pool, Mel suddenly stands, causing another tsunami in the hot tub.

"Don't get up," I say way too fast and loud, not daring to look anywhere near his huge, naked rolling mountain of flesh.

"See you around," Mel shouts as we grab our towels and practically sprint away. The last horrifying image I see, seared into my brain as if from a branding iron, is Mel's massive, hairy, fleshy planet of a butt descending into the bubbly water.

Hand in hand, like lovers on the lam, Amy and I pull up at the circus pool, now mostly obscured in shadow. I hear loud talk, occasional splashing, and whoops of laughter, but because of a sudden blinding purplish strobe light I can make out only vague body shapes.

"Let's go for a swim," I say to Amy. "Escape from Mel-zilla."

"I'm all in," Amy says, and plunges into the pool. I dive in right behind her and soon we surface diagonally across from the bottom of the waterslide. Gradually my eyes adjust to the dark and I'm able to squint through the strobe effect. I see twenty or so people around me, in and out of the pool, more if I count the steady flow who flash down the waterslide. Something about the way they look strikes me. More than a little taken back, I whisper to Amy, "Is the strobe light playing tricks on my eyes or is everybody here buck naked?"

"Nope. Your vision's fine. Everybody is nude. Except us."

"Whoa. Awkward."

"Little bit."

"Do you want to leave?" I ask.

"No. It's our vacation." Amy pauses. "Do you?"

"No. I mean, Mel freaked me out, but if we forget him, I like it here."

"I know. This pool is nice."

"OK, so, let's just, you know, try to ignore the, um, nudity and stuff."

"Not a problem for me," Amy says.

"Me either," I say.

"I'd actually like to try the waterslide."

"Me too."

"Let's do it."

"Keep your eyes straight ahead," Amy says.

"You too," I say.

We swim to the edge of the pool, lift ourselves out, and climb the ladder leading to the top of the waterslide. Amy goes first, takes a breath, kicks off, howling as she twists, turns, and flies like a happy seven-year-old down the slide. I follow, landing with a splash a few feet away from her. I surface, blink the water out of my eyes as a guy, tall, gray-haired, and naked, swims over to us and treads water in our wake. He is definitely checking us both out.

"You should go down the slide naked," he says. "You go much faster."

"Great, thanks for the tip," I say. "But we're good. Thank you though."

"I think we should try it," Amy says.

"Naked?"

"Yeah. Why not? Let's do it. When in Rome..."

"You go faster," naked guy says again. "It's a thrill."

"Huh," I say, looking at Amy, who grins at me. She seems to have forgotten that I have a phobia of being naked around others. Yes, I'm the guy who showers in the gym with my swimsuit on.

"Excuse me," the gray-haired guy says, waving at a naked woman standing at the side of the pool. He swims over and pulls himself up and out of the pool, his naked butt bouncing purple light at us from the strobe.

"You really want to go down the slide naked?" I say.

"Yeah. Maybe. I don't know. Would you?"

"Not tonight," I say. "It's too, uhh...chilly. And..."

I stop.

"Yeah, and?"

"I'm afraid of, you know, shrinkage."

"Shrinkage," Amy says.

"Yeah. With the water and the nervousness and the shyness there will be, like, major...junk shrinkage," I say, indicating my crotch.

"Major junk shrinkage? C'mon, honey, it's already a sausage fest," Amy says.

"Yes, but we're talking, like, *Vienna* sausage here," I say.

"Oh, yeah, we wouldn't want that."

"No," I say. "But I'll do the trapeze. Right now."

"Clothes on?"

"Clothes on."

"And you'll think about the waterslide, naked, shrinkage and all?"

"I will. But just once."

"That's all. Just once. Something to tell our grandkids."

I shoot her a look.

"Or not," she says.

* * *

For the rest of the week, we are, in the best way, accosted by undressed, totally exposed swingers. Naked, they join us at meals, in the gym, on the beach, at the pool, and at the nightly dance, each evening having a theme—Roaring Twenties, the Last Days of Disco, the Sound of the Sixties, Country Jamboree. Almost everyone we meet is friendly and fun, like there could be nothing more normal than doing the hustle or the "Achy Breaky" dance in your birthday suit. Almost no one, other than Mel, applies any pressure to join them in a three-way, a wife swap, or a ménage-a-whatever. I also point out to Amy a couple of characteristics that all the male swingers seem to share: they are over fifty, not bashful, and shave their genitals, offering up a stark white fleshy contrast to their matted, hairy backs and butts.

Funny what we can get used to. By the third day, completely content in my clothes, I pay almost no attention to the ever-present nudity and I allow myself to relax, undistracted by the naked bodies bulging and bumping around me. Every afternoon, Amy and I lounge by the pool tanning, reading, and, when the heat overcomes us, rolling into the water for a short dip to cool off. And every evening we whoosh down the waterslide at least once. The gray-haired guy, a treading-water fixture near the mouth of the slide, shakes his head as we emerge from underwater after careening down the slide and splashing into the pool, speaking through his smiling glossy white dentures, "You go much faster when you're naked."

The night before we check out, we decide to go for one last swim. We hold hands as we enter the pool area, as always, the only non-nudists in sight. We find a couple of lounge chairs and set up our stuff, taking our time, in no hurry, both of us secretly wishing that we could extend our vacation another few days at least.

"This has been great, just what the doctor ordered," I say.

"That's the naked truth," Amy says. "Ha."

"Ha-*ha*. Seriously, it's not that I've had any amazing insight or experienced any clarity, I just feel, I guess, calmer."

I sigh.

"I don't want this feeling to end."

"So don't let it."

I take that in.

To my left, someone shrieks and laughs. I peer in the direction of the sound and see two naked sixty-year-olds making out, their flabby rumpled bodies pressed close.

"I'm not sure I'll miss seeing that," I say.

"I don't know. It's kinda cute."

I turn back toward Amy. I gasp.

She's naked.

"What are you doing?" I say.

"Going down the waterslide," she says.

She grins and then starts to walk toward the edge of the pool.

"Wait," I say. "Don't."

She stops and tilts her head.

"Not without me," I say, and start to pull down my suit. I stop midway. "We're not coming back here next year, are we?"

"Not a chance."

I nod and drop my bathing suit down to my ankles.

Naked, Amy and I dive into the water. We climb out of the pool at the base of the waterslide's ladder and scramble up to the top of the slide. Amy sits, shivers, and pushes off down the slide. I'm right behind her, shooting down on my naked backside, picking up speed, scorching down that slide, fast as a missile. I plow into the water, sending an explosion of spray soaking every person and pool toy within twenty yards, including the gray-haired guy who dog paddles over to me.

"What a rush," I say.

"Told you," the gray-haired guy says.

"Go again?" Amy says, bobbing to the surface at my side.

"Absolutely," I say.

And we do, only slightly conscious of everyone's eyes checking out our bright white naked butts.

Well, *I'm* more than slightly conscious of them. Amy, God love her, seems to have shut everyone else out, shut out the world.

We go down the waterslide again, naked.

And again.

And again.

Preparing to fly down the waterslide for the fifth time, naked, I realize that this is why I came to Jamaica and why I stayed in this beautiful resort, the home of the hedonists, on Swingers Week.

I realize that to make it as a doctor, a plastic surgeon, a husband, maybe a dad someday—to make it in *life*—I have to first stand my ground and then give myself permission to let go.

That's what I have to do.

Let it all go.

And sometimes, just get naked.

24

Standing My Ground

The new patients change.

Just like that.

Gone are the ones who threatened, concerned, or traumatized me. Oh, on occasion, I get a call or take a consultation that sets off my inner alarm system, but for the most part, my patients fall into the range of humanity I happily refer to as *nice*.

And then, ever so slowly, I change. It begins when I consciously alter my perspective. Simply, I go back to basics. I remember the reason I decided to become a doctor in the first place—I want to help people. I embrace that. I remember my purpose, my joy, and let go of the fear.

As a plastic surgeon, I know that sometimes, most times, changing people means changing them literally, physically, adjusting the way they look. To that purpose, I become more selective, more discerning, and—my key adjustment—less desperate for business. I let go of the need to succeed, the frantic clamoring to bring in patients. The moment I do, incredibly, the more my business increases. As more patients seek my services, my confidence builds.

Then one day, I face a challenge that wallops me, forcing me to face a harsh reality: any patient may experience a catastrophic complication. And even if that complication isn't my fault, the patient is always my responsibility.

A woman in her sixties, call her Connie, comes to see me with her husband, Ray. Connie is a healthy, vibrant woman with soft blue eyes, a warm, easy smile, and long silver hair she wears braided halfway down her back. Connie wants a facelift.

"I have a close circle of friends," she says. "I'm the only one who hasn't had a facelift. They all look fifteen years younger. I have to keep up with them, you know?"

I laugh along with her and her husband and then I examine her. She definitely has some loose skin and jowls. I consider her a prime facelift candidate. We schedule her surgery, which, given her good health, I expect will be routine and straightforward.

I bring Connie into surgery and start her procedure. Working very meticulously, I cut around her ears and lift the skin off her face, cheeks, jaw line, and upper neck all the way down to the middle neck area. I remove any excess fat pockets, tighten the muscle area underneath, pull the skin back, and suture everything shut. Takes three hours. Typical.

I spend some time with her in the recovery room after she wakes up and look over my handiwork. Her jowls, gone. Neckline, tight. Modestly, I think she looks great. I congratulate her and tell her that after a few weeks she will soon look as young as her friends. She smiles, groggily. She'll be spending the night in the hospital and I promise to check on her in the morning.

I get in my car and start driving back to my office. Fifteen minutes later, I receive an urgent page from the nurse taking care of Connie. I call the nurse on my Bluetooth.

"It's about your patient Connie," the nurse says. "We think she's bleeding. We need you to come back and take a look at her."

"OK. I'm about fifteen minutes away," I say, craning my neck, searching for a safe place to turn around.

I then get a second page. "911." This message is urgent and cryptic. "Your patient's neck is filling up with blood. You need to come right now. "We need you *Stat*."

I weave into the middle lane, cut off a car, and, turning the steering wheel violently, whip into a U-turn, speed across all lanes, straighten out, and, facing the hospital, press my foot down on the gas. I nearly stand on the accelerator. My stomach flips and that foreboding feeling of nausea grips me. In my head I see the sudden, horrifying image of Connie's neck bloated with blood, closing off her airway, literally strangling her to death.

I blow through stop signs, my eyes darting through the windshield, hurtling and swerving around slow-moving vehicles, while simultaneously peeking at the rearview mirror, on the lookout for cops. *It won't matter if a cop comes after me*, I think. *I won't pull over. I'll keep going all the way to the hospital, pretending I have a police escort.*

"Come on, come *on*!" I say aloud, as if I can will my car to drive faster, whip it to arrive at the hospital quicker. I whack the steering wheel with my palms, praying that I will reach Connie before it's too late.

After only ten minutes—five minutes less than it would take driving the speed limit—I screech to a stop at the hospital's automatic front double doors, rush out of the car, and toss my keys to the dozing and startled valet parking attendant. I race inside, breaking into a full-on sprint. I bolt past the bank of elevators, throw my shoulder into the door leading to the staircase, and fly up the stairs, taking two, then three at a time. I skid across the second-floor landing, nearly fall, bang through the door, and run across the second-floor lobby, careen past the nurses' station, take a wide turn around the corner, and charge into Connie's room. Panting, I lean over for a second to catch my breath while glancing at the human form in the hospital bed. Connie, I assume. I hesitate because the person lying in the bed bears little resemblance to Connie.

This person looks like Jabba the Hut.

Her neck, filled with blood, has expanded to four times its normal size. Scattered around the room I recognize members of Connie's family. Behind me, Connie's husband, Ray, stands, bent over, his face white, his fists balled up and resting on his knees.

"Doctor Youn, thank you for coming," he says. "What's happened to her?"

Ray lifts his head and searches my face for something, an answer, some assurance, some hope. I'm breathing too hard to respond. A nurse steps in front of him, blocking him from my vision, and looking from me back to Connie and her gigantic neck, she whispers frantically, "What do we do? I've never seen anything like this. Tell me what to do."

I breathe in, out. "Get me a pair of scissors."

The nurse freezes.

"Now. Get me some scissors. *Run!*"

I whip around to the medical supply cabinet, pull open a drawer, rummage around, find a pair of gloves, and pull them on.

"Scissors!" I scream to the room, to no one.

In seconds, with all sound crashing into a muffled mash-up of shouting, shoes squeaking on the floor, monitors beeping, instruments scraping, indeterminate humming and murmuring, the nurse hands me the scissors, and in street clothes, no time for scrubs or scrubbing up, no thought of sterilization, my thinking reduced to one sentence blinking in oversized blazing neon letters, *I have to save Connie's life*, I press her face and shoulder near her neckline, hard, determine that she's still significantly numb from the amount of anesthetic she's taken in, and with the scissors, I cut away all the sutures I put in place only hours ago. I once again lift Connie's skin, and using only my gloved hands, I dig into her open neck and scoop out a fistful of gelatinous blood. A nurse shoves a paper towel beneath my fingers and I drop the blood onto it. I go back inside Connie's neck again and again, digging out huge pulsating crimson globs, dropping them, plop, onto the paper towel.

"I'm so sorry about this," I say to Connie. "I know it hurts, but I have to do this. I'm so sorry."

"What the *hell* is going on?" Ray says, his voice broken and distant.

I don't answer. I continue scooping out chunks of blood, handfuls of blood, pouring it all onto the pile of accumulating paper towels. And then, very gradually, Connie's swollen, pumpkin-sized neck begins to deflate. I see, though, that a small artery continues to bleed. I press on it with my finger.

"Call the OR," I say to the nurse hovering over my shoulder, her main concern managing the bloody paper towels. "We have to get her down there right now. As in *right now.*"

As the nurse stretches for the phone on the wall, I turn back to Connie, trying to sound as comforting and natural as possible, knowing how ridiculous I look and sound, my voice quavering, my blue dress shirt drenched with an island of her blood, but seeing, thankfully, that her neck continues to deflate.

"OK, we're good, getting there. How you doing? You OK?"

"I think so," she says. "This is pretty freaking scary."

"I know. It's really unusual. Extremely rare. Are you hurting at all?"

"No. I'm a little uncomfortable, but actually, I feel a lot better right now than I did before."

"I'm really sorry this happened to you. Such a freak thing. Basically, one of the clots fell off one of your arteries. I had to do all this so you wouldn't, well, *choke.*" I whirl back toward the nurse, my finger still pressed on the artery inside Connie's neck. "How are we doing with that OR?"

"They're ready," the nurse says. "They said bring her right down."

For the next hour, I fall into some altered state, seeing myself from outside my body—wheeling Connie to the OR, Ray trailing behind, his face ashen, the sound of his voice skimming past me, assaulting me with indecipherable questions, peppered with fear and disbelief; the hot lights of the OR bearing down, my finger still attached to the artery in Connie's neck, refusing to let go, noticing, though, that much of the bleeding has stopped; putting Connie under heavy anesthetic again, and I'm operating, again, washing away all the blood that remains built up in her neck; and then I'm suturing her for the second time and suddenly, Connie, her face battered, a punched-out purple mess, but alive, sleeping in her hospital room as I stand outside in the hall trying to explain everything to Ray and, in some way, to myself.

"I'm sorry you had to see that," I say, shaking my head, realizing that all I seem to do is apologize.

"It was like a slasher film," Ray says. "Gory as hell."

"I know. I'm sorry," I say, apologizing yet again. "What happened was really unusual. But if we had waited even another few minutes, her airway was closing off...I don't want to go there."

"You saved her life," Ray says.

"Well, I..."

Ray hugs me.

"Thank you," he says, his arms wrapped around me, his cheeks wet with tears pressing into mine.

"She's going to look bad for a while," I say, as we break apart. "Be prepared."

"For how long?"

"Three weeks. Maybe a month."

"And then?"

"Oh, she'll be fine." And then I smile. "She's gonna look just as good as her friends."

I'm guessing at the time frame, but I know I'm right about the result.

A month later, Connie comes to my office for her follow-up.

She looks great and she couldn't be happier.

She looks and feels fifteen years younger.

Now, in the hospital, after Ray leaves, I head into a washroom to clean up before I head home. Over my shoulder, I see the nurse who did such amazing work managing the globs of blood I placed on paper towels, standing in the doorway.

"I've never seen anything like that," she says.

"Me neither," I say, with a half-smile. "I've never had anyone bleed like that."

"What you did..." the nurse says, shaking her head.

"Well, if that ever happens again and I'm not around, feel free to cut out all the stitches and do what you have to do."

"First off, there's no way I'd be able to cut out your stitches," the nurse says.

I shrug.

"You saved her life," the nurse says.

This is the second time someone has said that to me within ten minutes.

"Allow me to shake your hand," and as I do the nurse says, "It's an honor to work with you, Doctor Youn."

And that's when I realize, finally, that I am a doctor.

The doctor I have always wanted to be.

* * *

Playing God.

I see doctors who become holier than thou, who think they're God—lording over their patients, nurses, staff, even hospital administrators.

Of course, I've seen doctors who've played God with *me*.

I don't play God.

I wouldn't dare.

Because I need God.

I need God to watch over me, to guide me, to help me, to keep me sane and my patients safe.

Whenever I consult a patient for a procedure, inevitably the patient will ask, "What's the worst that can happen to me? Describe the worst-case scenario." I always respond, "Well, technically, you could die."

I let that sink in.

I follow that up with, "The chances are small, tiny, less than the chance of you getting in a car accident on the way home and dying. But the chances are not zero."

It's out of my hands, I want to tell my patients. *It's up to God. But I'm always hoping—praying—that God will stand beside me in your surgery. So far, every time, I've felt His presence, so I think we're going to be all right.*

* * *

A woman, call her Betsy, comes to see me. Betsy is in her early sixties and horribly unhealthy. She walks with a cane, each step she takes slow and painful. It hurts to watch her walk. Betsy has undergone a quadruple bypass, survived renal cancer, and weighs 240 pounds, even though she has lost 150 pounds after a recent gastric bypass surgery. She also has a history of diabetes, depression, and anxiety disorder, leading me to believe she may be bipolar. She currently takes twenty different medications a day. She is, what we call in the medical profession, a train wreck.

Huffing, her face pulsing red, she lowers herself into a chair and then takes a count of twenty to catch her breath. She looks me over. Her lips tremble. I think she is about to cry.

"You're my last hope," Betsy says. "Everybody else has turned me down. Will you help me?"

I go blank.

And then that loud warning buzzer in my head bleats.

Turn her down, turn her down, turn her down!

She sniffs. I hand her a tissue and slide the box next to her elbow.

"I've seen a dozen other surgeons," she says. "They all sent me away."

Did I mention that her complexion is raw and cratered and inflamed; she's taking blood-thinning pills, has terrible hypertension, and is on multiple psychiatric medications?

She's too high risk. There's no point in even talking to her. Turn her down!

I can't.

"So," I say, "tell me what's going on."

Betsy clears her throat, sighs, and lets it all out, whoosh, in one frantic breath. "I had the surgery and lost all this weight and then I had a tummy tuck and it went wrong. Everything fell apart, like, everything fell *apart*. I developed a terrible infection and I was in the hospital on IV antibiotics for, like, two months. I went to rehab afterward but it didn't really help. Now my tummy is completely destroyed. I have constant, chronic, terrible pain. I can barely walk. I have this horrible, disgusting scar tissue. I'm disabled, see? I can't do anything."

She stops to catch her breath.

She is a medical disaster and a major postsurgical complication waiting to happen.

Send her away. Turn her down.

Betsy snatches a tissue from the box, blows her nose, honks, fights to keep from bursting into tears.

"Can you continue?" I ask her.

She nods. "At first I thought the tummy tuck was OK, but two days after the surgery, I got an infection and huge parts of my stomach turned *black*."

"Turned black?" I say and feel myself frown.

"I kept going back to have the plastic surgeon cut out the dead tissue. And that's when I got some kind of staph infection or flesh-eating bacteria."

"Holy cow," I say, amazed she's still alive.

"It's been, like, five months now and there's a huge chunk gone from my tummy and the whole area just hurts constantly."

OK, I think, *there is absolutely no way I'm operating on this woman. She's way too high risk. For a start, I'd have to take her off the blood thinners, but then she could get blood clots and we know how dangerous that can be. And with her history of diabetes, cancer, and infection, she could develop terrible healing problems. No-brainer. A definite no.*

I nod at her stomach. "Do you mind if I take a look?"

She changes into a gown, returns, and I examine her abdomen. To begin with, her stomach protrudes, hangs over her waist like a massive beer belly. The stomach area itself is both horribly scarred and socked in. I look further and see a kind of trench as well as charred skin, almost as if Betsy is a burn patient. It's basically a mess.

Betsy grips the tip of her cane. "I know. It's disgusting. I can barely walk. I'm in constant pain. I can't play with my grandkids. My husband won't even look at me."

Betsy begins sobbing uncontrollably.

"I'm...deformed," she sputters between sobs. "I have no life."

This is a nightmare. I would be taking a huge risk. There are so many potential complications. She could die and it would be all on my watch. Fifteen other doctors turned her down!

"Please, Doctor Youn," Betsy says, her eyes soaked with tears. "You're my last hope. I have nowhere else to go. Please help me."

Turn!

Her!

Down!

"I can't," I say, swallowing. "I just can't say no to you."

"You'll help me?"

"I will."

"Oh, my God, thank you."

Betsy lowers her head and cries even harder.

I take her hands.

And now the strange part.

I know I'm not alone.

I actually feel God telling me to help her.

OK, right, I know, to some of you that may sound weird and crazy and over the edge and...fill in the blank.

But I'm totally serious. I *feel* God telling me to help her.

How?

I just do.

I also feel strangely calm and composed.

I know that I have to help this woman and that it will be OK, despite her litany of woes and illnesses and messed-up surgeries and the sheer odds stacked against her, almost guaranteeing some kind of deadly complication. A complication that I'll be held responsible for. But I'm no longer worried about me. This is bigger than me.

It is crazy, otherworldly, surreal...because I feel as if I've been—

Chosen.

To help her.

It feels like more than the right thing.

It feels like the only thing.

I know I *have* to do it.

God is telling me that this woman needs my help.

"My insurance," Betsy mumbles. "I don't know how much, if anything, it will cover...."

"We'll submit it," I say. "Whatever it covers, great. But even if it doesn't cover anything, don't worry. It's fine. It doesn't matter. I'm not gonna charge you."

"I don't know what to say," Betsy says, and she cries louder, her sobs rising to an unprecedented level of volume and intensity.

Finally, she's able to calm herself and I say, "No promises, OK?"

"I know," she says. "No promises."

* * *

The night before Betsy's surgery, I pray.

I ask God to please help me to help Betsy. I thank Him for my experience and my training and my skill as a surgeon and I pray for Him to watch over Betsy during the operation and to please, *please*, keep any complications to a minimum.

And then I try to sleep.

I fail.

It's funny, this whole idea of playing God.

Doctors don't have to play God, because patients routinely put them, especially surgeons, in that position. I always remind myself that in fact it's very much the opposite. Not only am I not God nor should I play God, but I need God to help me.

Feeling at peace, I drift off to sleep.

During Betsy's surgery, which takes four hours, I not only feel God's presence the whole time, but I feel His hands guiding me. I complete the procedure, correcting Betsy's tummy tuck, cleaning it up, smoothing it out, without a hitch. She recovers without a hint of a complication. I follow up with her three weeks later—everything looks good—and a month after that, she arrives in my office, walking without a cane, holding a carrot cake she's baked for me.

"So nice of you," I say. "Thank you."

"Kind of the least I could do for saving my life."

Her bottom lip trembles.

"Yesterday I played with my granddaughter and for the first time in two years, I could hold her in my lap."

Her eyes well up.

"What made you do it?"

I look at her. "I don't know what you mean. Do what?"

"Take a chance on me. Take the risk that nobody else would."

"I don't know," I say. "I just knew I had to. I had faith that I was meant to do it and everything would be all right."

"Well, I'll never be able to adequately thank you," she says, shaking her head at the carrot cake, full payment for the procedure since her insurance company turned her down. It doesn't matter. I'm sure the carrot cake is delicious, although I have a policy to never eat anything baked by patients.

"Some doctors..." Betsy says, removing the wrapping from the carrot cake and cutting herself a piece. She offers me a slice.

I smile, shake my head, and mouth *Later*.

"Especially these surgeons," Betsy says again, her cheeks puffed out with carrot cake, "are so high and mighty. They think they're God. Not you."

"No," I say. "I don't think I'm God. Far from it."

What the hell.

I reach over and grab a slice of that carrot cake.

It *is* delicious.

"I'm just a doctor," I say.

Acknowledgments
for Anthony Youn, M.D.

First and foremost, thank you to God for blessing me and my family beyond our wildest dreams. Great is Thy faithfulness.

To Amy, my wife and the woman of my dreams. Thank you for always being supportive of my many projects. I love you so much. Looking forward to many more adventures as we grow old together.

To Mom and Dad. Thank you for your unconditional love and encouragement. I hope you really enjoyed this one. Thank you for letting me tell your story.

To Alan Eisenstock. We did it again, my friend. I wouldn't want to tell my story with anyone else.

To Wendy Sherman. My literary agent, my friend, and my trusted advisor. Thank you for believing in me and believing in *Playing God*. Onward!

To Heather King, Debra Englander, and everyone at Post Hill Press. I am beyond delighted that you chose to publish this book. It's an honor to be one of your authors.

To Dr. Brian Smith. I wouldn't be a three-time-published author without you. Thank you for your advice, contributions, and friendship.

To Lisa and Mike, Jim and Py. Thank you for being my biggest cheerleaders. Your support means the world to me.

To David Henry Sterry. Thank you for your valuable input on this book.

To my friends and family who have bought my books, including my awesome cousins and the gang from Greenville. There are too many of you to name, and I fear I would inadvertently leave someone out. Thank you for supporting me and sharing my books with others. I value your friendships more than you know.

To JJ, Karl, and the Mindshare Community. Thank you for having my back. It's an honor to be one of you.

To the doctors who trained me and the patients who educated me. I hope these stories do justice to everything you've done to make me the doctor I am today.

To my employees at YOUN Plastic Surgery and the staff at my local hospital (nurses, PAs, surgical techs, and others). Thank you for helping me care for my patients and supporting me in my creative endeavors. I couldn't be who I am today without your help.

To my patients, past and present. Thank you for trusting in me to be your physician. It's an honor and a privilege I do not take for granted.

To my followers and friends on social media (Instagram, Facebook, YouTube, and Twitter). Thank you for spending your time with me and your hard-earned money on my books and products. I couldn't do this without your daily support and interaction! I look forward to hearing what you think of this book!

Finally, to D and G. You mean everything to me. Do your best, be respectful and kind, and love with reckless abandon. I am always so proud of you.

Acknowledgments for Alan Eisenstock

Thanks once again to Tony. You are a dynamo, as a doctor, coauthor, and friend. I feed off your never-say-die spirit.

Thanks to Wendy Sherman for finding the perfect home for *Playing God*.

Thanks to everyone at Post Hill Press for all your support.

Thanks to Anthony Mattero. The best.

Thanks to my literary lifeline, David Ritz.

Thanks to my posse—Madeline and Phil Schwarzman, Sue Pomerantz and George Weinberger, Susan Baskin and Richard Gerwitz, Kathy Montgomery and Jeff Chester, Linda Nussbaum, Ed Feinstein.

Thanks to my family—Jim Eisenstock, Jay Eisenstock, Loretta Barrabee, Lorraine, Linda, Diane, Alan, Chris, Ben, Nate, and, always, Brian.

Jonah, Kiva, and Randy, you fill me up every day, thank you for everything, always.

Z, GG, and Snickers, thank you forever.

Finally, thanks to Bobbie, LOML, you are my world.

About the Authors

Anthony Youn, M.D. is known as America's Holistic Beauty Doc™ and one of the country's most recognized plastic surgeons. He is the host of a popular podcast, *The Holistic Plastic Surgery Show*. Dr. Youn is also the author of *In Stitches*, his critically acclaimed and award-winning memoir of becoming a doctor (Gallery Books/Simon & Schuster, 2011), and *The Age Fix: A Leading Plastic Surgeon Reveals How To Really Look Ten Years Younger* (Grand Central Life & Style/Hachette, 2016). The latter was adapted into a successful public television special which has been viewed by millions. Dr. Youn is also a regular expert on *The Rachael Ray Show, The Dr. Oz Show, The Doctors*, and many more national television programs. Named a "Top Plastic Surgeon" by *U.S. News and World Report, Town & Country*, and *Harper's Bazaar*, Dr. Youn is a member of the American Society of Plastic Surgeons (ASPS), the American Society for Aesthetic Plastic Surgery (ASAPS), and a fellow of the American College of Surgeons. He is an Assistant Professor of Surgery at the Oakland University William Beaumont School of Medicine.

Alan Eisenstock is the author of seventeen books, most recently *Love Thy Neighbor: A Muslim Doctor's Struggle for Home in Rural America* (Convergent Books), written with Dr. Ayaz Virji. He lives in Pacific Palisades, California.